Other Books Available from Broken Sword Publications

Alcohol Soaked & Nicotine Stained

Demon in the Mirror

AmeriKKKan Stories

¡Ban This! The BSP Anthology of Chican@ Literature

Josh Divine's Ducktown

Lowriting: Shots, Rides & Stories from the Chicano Soul

#FuckCancer

The True Story of How Robert the Bold Kicked Cancer's Ass

by Robert Flores

Edited by Santino J. Rivera

Foreword by Gustavo Arellano

Photographs by Art Meza

Broken Sword Publications

Saint Augustine, Fla

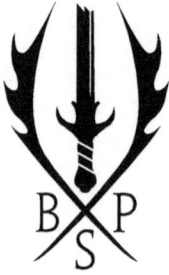

Broken Sword Publications

Saint Augustine, Florida, USA

First Printing August 2015

Cover photography and interior photos by Art Meza aka @Chicano_Soul, www.chicanosoul.net

Other photos provided by Robert Flores.

Book design and layout by Josh Divine, www.joshdivine.com

Special thanks to Lisa Rivera, Dolores D. Avila and

Nelly Guajardo for proofreading services.

Broken Sword Publications, LLC

Web: www.brokenswordpublications.com

Store: bsp.bigcartel.com

E-Mail: mail@brokenswordpublications.com

Twitter: @brokenswordpub

IG: @BrokenSwordPublications

ISBN 978-0-9896313-2-7

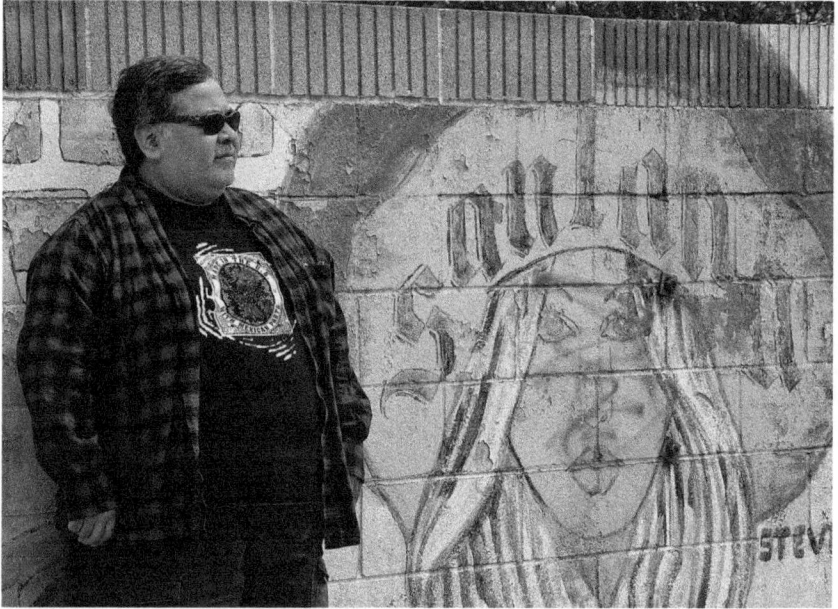

I dedicate this to my family. For my Mom, Hortense R. Flores, for raising me right, for always believing in me, trusting me, praying for me and taking care of me. For Kevin, my brother, I am your older brother but I felt you watching over me, every day, cooking my meals and picking me up from so many appointments. For my sister, Denise, for helping me along the way and to Jeff, worried about his big brother, and never losing faith in me.

Thank you.

Robert Flores, May 17, 2015
Santa Ana, California

Contents

Foreword: Behold the Butcher, Cancer Killer

By Gustavo Arellano

We call him the Butcher, and not just because Robert Flores is a carnicero by trade and has done so for more than 35 years. Bobby's as sharp as the knives he uses for a living—the knowledge of his skills, his humor, the hooks and crosses he unleashes whenever my friends and cousins go through a boxing session at the Mexiclan Dojo. I've never heard him play the sax or drive the VW bug in his garage, two hobbies he's yet to share with us, but I'm sure he does the two with an exacting verve as only someone who slices, chops, saws, and eviscerates for a living can do.

And now, I'm proud to say he's also a sharp author as well. F*ck Cancer! is an awesome, unsparing, hilarious, touching look into the life of not just a cancer survivor, but a cancer killer. You have to possess the mindset of a meatman to make it through the hell that is Stage 4 colon cancer: methodical, precise, unsparing, prepared for the gore and blood that follows when it confronts you. It's a disease that beats down almost everyone, especially when it's at the final stage before it's ready to turn you into a carcass. But the Butcher prevailed—and now wants to tell his survival tale for the world, a story I'm proud to promote and even play a small part in.

I can't even remember anymore the first time Robert and I met. He knew me long before I knew him, since Bobby read my stuff in the OC Weekly for years before we spoke a word to each other. Maybe it was on Twitter, where he sent me enough nice things for me to follow him, then posted enough hilarity for me to retweet incessantly. Maybe it was via Facebook, which says we've been amigos since October 2011. Maybe it was in—of all places—the Cypress Park Library in Los Angeles, home to one of the coolest librarians around, so cool that his Lowriting: Shots, Rides and Stories from the Chicano Soul featured entries by both Robert and I (you can buy the book through the publisher of this book, Broken Sword Publications—what, you don't think we shamelessly cross-promote our stuff here?)

Truth is, I forgot when I finally had the pleasure of knowing Robert, and I really don't give a fuck: Bobby is my brother now, and it feels like we've known each other forever. I think we immediately got along because we shared the same love of food, the same hatred of vendido politicians, and the same commitment to raise DESMADRE. I forgave him that he attended Mater Dei High School, which is as famous for its pedophile priests as it is for its powerhouse prep football and basketball programs; he looked past the fact that I'm from Anaheim, and he's from big, bad SanTana.

We immediately hit it off, and I introduced him to my inner circle, one member who—talk about fate—had worked with Bobby at a supermarket a decade earlier. But in those first couple of meetings, I didn't know he was battling for his life. The remarkable thing about the Butcher is that any despair he may have is quickly leveled by his determination and optimism, so that Butcher's public face is that of a typical middle-aged chingón who wants nothing more than a beer, a burger and a football game on the screen to call it a night. As you'll read in these pages, he definitely went through highs and lows, but NEVER gave up. I always tell young students that the way through life is always forward—you can slow down, but never stop, and NEVER go back. In Butcher's case, he didn't just keep going forward: he cut down the shitstorm of life.

**

I come from a family of cancer survivors—my dad had testicular cancer, while Mami beat back breast cancer. I had one of my OC Weekly photographers pass away from the same cancer that struck Robert (you'll read more about him soon). It's a vicious thing that lays waste to the strongest people—and it's absolutely taboo to talk about it in Mexican society. We're supposed to face it stoically, without drawing attention to ourselves. But that does nothing to help others, or the sufferer himself.

F*ck Cancer! is not just the latest entry in the lengthy bookshelf of cancer literature; it also very much belongs in Chicano Studies classrooms. Because in the Butcher, you find everything we want our community to turn into: a fighter. A survivor. Someone who's proud of where they're from. Brown and down. And a pioneer: Robert is brave enough to tell his story, brave enough to become a writer despite being in his mid-50s and never having written a "professional" story, let alone a full-length book. May this book inspire people who want to be writers but are afraid to do so…to do so. May the Butcher inspire other cancer survivors—especially raza—to tell their stories. May F*ck Cancer! give families the courage to talk about this subject. May this book top the New York Times bestseller list…yeah right, they still think the only "Hispanic" writer worth covering is Richard Rodriguez.

But most of all, may anyone who read F*ck Cancer! come away inspired by the Butcher to do something with their lives. Because if this man looked death in the face, took its scythe, and chopped it down could do it, then so can you.

Gustavo Arellano is editor of OC Weekly, author of the syndicated column ¡Ask a Mexican! and consulting producer on FOX's animated show, Bordertown.

Introduction: Fucking Cancer and Documenting the Process

By Santino J. Rivera

How, exactly, do you fuck cancer? It's a good question and one that's been on my mind for as long as I've seen the phrase "fuck cancer" on the web, which, by the way, is as popular now as it was when I saw it start to surface years ago. It's a hashtag now, used on every social media medium that exists: #fuckcancer. People like saying it and why shouldn't they? It gives you a little bit of power over something that terrifies even the most bold.

Is it dismissive? Authoritative? Punitive? Kinky?! You decide. That's the thing with the word 'fuck' – it has as many interpretations as it does inflections. Which brings me to my point: what is this book about?

No doubt, if you picked it up you are curious and want to know how Robert Flores kicked cancer's ass and why he might use such a brazen title. Truth be told, this book has been in the works for some time and I have to apologize for its tardiness but every book has a life of its own and this one took extra special care to get it right.

One thing that I try and do is to create books that would otherwise never see print. I enjoy making books that the mainstream publishing world either scoffs at or completely ignores. That means taking a risk. I also like to publish stuff that I would like to read. So, that, in essence, is what this is.

#FuckCancer is the true account of how my friend, Robert Flores, overcame the odds and beat cancer. And as he will tell you, himself, he didn't just beat cancer, he kicked its ass.

You might remember Robert (a proud Santana, Califas native) from his killer poem in Lowriting: Shots, Rides & Stories from the Chicano Soul. The poem, "Take A Little Trip With Me," which continues to blow people away every time Robert reads it. It comes straight from the heart of a man who faced his own Goliath, and won.

This book details the journey that he went on when this character that we call Cancer, decided to knock on his door one day, and challenge him to a fight. Never one to shy away from a challenge, Robert "The Bold" Flores AKA "Bobby The Butcher" said,   "Bring it on!"

A quick note about Robert's nicknames; as the title of the book suggests, he is "Robert The Bold." This nickname automatically made me think of royalty and a few other things, including Erik The Red, who was a Viking explorer with a big beard…when I first started talking to Robert the Bold, he had a similar beard.

"Robert The Bold" comes from Robert's barhopping days where a free shirt was offered for every 100th 32-ounce draft beer tankard consumed. When you reached 100, you got a tankard shirt and your name on the wall. Robert chose "Robert The Bold." He has 10 shirts. 'Nuff said.

The name stuck. It has a great ring to it and what better way to kick the shit out of cancer than with an epic name like "Robert The Bold"? Right.

Robert is also known as "Bobby The Butcher," and as you will read, he is a skilled meat cutter by trade. He's also a boxing fan and "the butcher" nickname was also appropriate for kicking cancer's ass. Seriously, Cancer had no chance.

A few years ago, when Robert was diagnosed with stage 4 colon cancer, he sought a mentor and found no one. There was nowhere for him to turn and no one to ask questions of or hear about what it was like to go through something like this, so he took matters into his own hands and began to blog about his experience online. Little did he know that he was writing a book…

Years ago now, I worked in the medical field as an EMT and trained as a firefighter. I know all too well what cancer looks like and it scares the shit out of me. It scares the shit out of everyone.

The "Big C," as it's known in some circles, is such a badass that when you hear the word you tend to think of two things: life and death. But one thing is for sure, everyone gets quiet.

Want to quiet a room up in a hurry? Talk about cancer and watch everyone shut the fuck up. It has that kind of stigma to it and that's wrong – it's a showstopper.

Some of the things that I know about medicine, I take for granted. I know that getting diagnosed with stage 4 cancer is grim news to say the least and you will find many that will call it a death sentence. I know that watching people waste away in nursing homes from their chemo and radiation treatments is painful in itself, if not life-changing. I also know that each cancer story is different. This is Robert's.

When Robert was first diagnosed he reached out online and found a community of support he was not expecting. True, it was not the mentor he was looking for, but it was a community of support that followed him every step of the way and still continues to this day.

As he endured his own personal Hell, he wrote about it on his blog. He put these things in his own voice and wrote from the heart. It was engaging. It dawned on me that his story – his personal experience with this demon, Cancer – was something that other people should hear.

In my experience most people don't write about this kind of stuff because it's too painful. Add to that the difficulty of documenting it while enduring it. Most people are not gonna share that kind of pain by choice with strangers, much less their own circle. And they're not going to detail what it's like to go through that kind of Hell because it's a special kind of Hell and one that is usually solitary.

When I went to the bookstore to do some research and check out what kind of books they had on cancer I was surprised to find that the shelves mostly consisted of books written by doctors and celebrities. There were also cookbooks and medical journals and a whole assortment of topics ranging from holistic medicine techniques, to spiritual manuals. But what was missing was a book by a regular person that said, "Hey! This is what's it's like to have cancer and go through chemo and radiation! No fluff or bullshit!"

For me, that's what is lacking in the medical book industry; books by regular folks and their experiences and wisdom. Why? Because when you get diagnosed with something life-threatening your mind goes a million miles an hour and all you want to do is talk with someone who has been through it and ask them the hard questions.

Yet, very often, all you find is cold waiting rooms, smiling nurses, perpetually late doctors, pamphlets in Greek, impersonal online forums and a shitload of bad info via a Google search.

Add to that, that there are practically ZERO Brown or Black voices detailing their experiences with these kinds of things in book form. I always get a kick (and not a haha one) out of visiting the "Hispanic" section of any bookstore and finding the same four or five books there, if that. There are NONE in the medical section. Why?

How is it that we can be leaders in statistics with things like diabetes and certain kinds of cancer yet there are no accounts of those experiences? Hence, just like with my other books, I sought to change that.

Robert chose the popular phrase "fuck cancer" as his mantra early on. Like a Shaolin Buddhist monk, he used it to motivate him to kick cancer's ass. And he did, which is amazing when you take everything into account.

The phrase "fuck cancer" is so popular, in fact, that I questioned naming the book that but then this story is not everyone's. This is the story of "Robert the Bold." And it just fits his story so well.

As he will tell you, Robert Flores lives in Santana, works in Santana, drinks in Santana…and he kicked Cancer's ass in Santana, literally. This is the story of a Chicano who took it upon himself to kick the shit out of cancer and document it so that it might help other people someday. And I wanted to preserve that because I believe it's important.

There are a couple of things I need to mention about the book before you venture on. First, this is not a traditional medical book. I don't do traditional books (duh!). Robert is not a conventional writer either – he blogged about his experiences in as honest a way as he could and he put it all on the line. He did all of this without any prior knowledge that any of it would be turned into a book so this is pure, raw experience with my editing for clarity.

You will read about exactly what he went through, no punches pulled, and for that he is "Robert the Bold." It's not easy putting these kinds of things into print (as you will read). I feel it's important to note that this book was written diary-style and on-line via Robert's Tumblr.

The book is as close as I could get to what he put in his blog over the span of a few years. I wanted to preserve his voice as much as possible and I wanted you to read these things as I did, in the same order that I did.

That said; some of the events are out of order as he remembers things or goes through them, so there may be a little bit of confusion from time to time. I have included a timeline so that you can see where he started and ended up.

I would like to thank author Gustavo Arellano of Taco USA, Ask A Mexican, and soon to be hit cartoon, Border Town, for lending his voice to this book, for the foreword. Gus is Robert's friend and he has a unique perspective into the kicking of cancer's ass, as you will read about.

I also want to thank photographer, Art Meza, who is a great friend of mine and Robert's. Art lent his photographic talents here so that we could capture Robert with his lens.

Okay, I've babbled on long enough. Are you ready to take another trip with the nerd con cuatro ojos? Rally the homies and get ready to kick Cancer's ass. This time it's personal.

Fuck Cancer!

#FuckCancer Timeline

December 2011 – Diagnosed with colorectal cancer

January 2012 - Start six chemotherapy treatments

March 2012 – Start 28 Radiation treatments

July 2012 – Surgery

December 2012 – Start 12 chemotherapy treatments

June 2013 – Cancer fee

"You never know how strong you are, until being strong is your only choice."

- Bob Marley

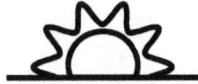

Part I: The Beginning

The Beginning

I don't know how I got cancer. Did I eat too much red meat? Did I not drink enough water? Too much fast food? Or was I just genetically predisposed to get it? The luck of the draw I suppose.

Both my parents have had cancer.

My Mom survived breast cancer. My Dad had three different types of cancer, the third one, no, actually the fourth one, killed him.

What I do know is that by the time my doctor found out about my own cancer, I had a 13-centimeter long tumor that ran from my colon along my sphincter to my rectum and actually came out through the skin of my left butt cheek. It was so low on my body that I didn't have any indication that it was something serious, such as loss of appetite or lack of energy. I just kept working hard as usual and playing hard as well.

Eventually, I went to my doctor thinking I probably had

hemorrhoids and a cyst. That was the beginning of my dance with the devil.

Let me rewind a little.

I was born in 1959 to Robert and Hortense Flores in Santa Ana, California. My Dad was also born in Santa Ana and my Mom was born and grew up in Stanton, California. I am the oldest of four children. I have a sister, Denise and two brothers, Kevin and Jeffrey. Our childhood was so normal that we probably thought we were White – assimilation back then was all the rage.

My Mom went to school in Anaheim in the mid-1930s. Back then you were punished physically if you spoke one word of Spanish. So, we weren't really taught a second language growing up, but I was able to pick up enough to survive as I grew older.

We went on month-long camping vacations during the summer; Yellowstone and Canada one summer and all the way down to Mexico City and the state of Guanajuato another.

I did well in school. Everything was hunky-dory, peachy keen. Then, when I was 13-years-old, my parents divorced and everyone's world changed. Through the strength of my Mom, we survived. I became a meat cutter. It's been my only job and I've been working in butcher shops since I was 17.

My brothers and sister all worked their way through college. When I was around 35 I met someone and got married, the relationship and marriage lasted about ten years.

A pretty normal life.

Until now.

My Chemo Starts Wednesday – December 14, 2012 09:12 P.M.

Finally, I will start my Chemo treatment. I'm at the same time looking forward to it and not looking forward to it. Ha! But this is the final stage to getting rid of this cancer.

I will have six sessions every two weeks. Every week I will also have a two-hour treatment of Erbitux[1]; this drug will starve the cancer of blood and oxygen.

Yay!

Fuck cancer.

Chemo is like being on a roller coaster; once you get on you can't get off. There are ups and downs. The downs are bad – very bad. That's why I'm starting this blog – to let you all know what it's really like. So if you have a weak stomach I advise you not to read this. This won't be easy for me to write while I go through this.

As most of you know, I have already had chemo and radiation done, so I'm an experienced chemo warrior.

You have to take the good with the bad. I have mostly just posted pictures of my culinary exploits, aka "the good."

This will be different.

---

1 Erbitux (cetuximab) is a cancer medication that interferes with the growth of cancer cells and slows their growth and spread in the body.

I will lose my appetite. I will not want to write anything because I will not have the strength to think clearly. I will be on all kinds of drugs.

If I am able to I will also write about some of my experiences since I was diagnosed with cancer. It's been a year now. December 12th to be exact.

I've been through a lot.

A lot-a lot.

So bear with me. This should be an interesting ride to say the least.

I'm No Expert on Guns but... – December 14, 2012, 10:18 P.M.

I own three guns; a high powered .223 rifle, a 9mm Sig Sauer and a .45 Para Ordinance, but I'm no expert. In fact, I haven't shot a gun since 9/11.

Before 9/11 I used to go out to the desert with my buddies from work. They would invite me to go out camping and shooting out past the Marine Corps Air Ground Combat Center (MCAGCC), aka 29 Palms, in southern San Bernardino County, California.

They found a great place to shoot that bordered the back edge of the base – a lot of rock formations they dubbed the "dome." Perfect shelter. It was pretty far from the main road and they had motorcycles and an ATV that I rode.

Good times.

They taught me how to shoot and take care of my guns. Safety first, always! So I bought my first gun, the Sig. Nice but my favorite is the .45. Power!

Along with shooting targets, my friends made homemade bombs; gun powder, fuses, gasoline...BOOM! High octane fun in the great beyond.

We also had a lot of food and beer of course. You go out there for a few days to unwind. It was about a four hour drive from Orange County.

I remember one time, we drove out there and were so excited to shoot off some rounds, that as soon as we parked, we shot off our guns. Then, we heard someone else shoot some rounds to let us know where they were. Imagine you drive out to BFE, somewhere where you've never seen a soul ...POW! POW! POW! Then you hear: POW! POW!

POW! And it wasn't an echo.

We could hardly sleep.

No one was ever injured from our shooting but a friend did die out there. We had another spot that was out by Adelanto – this one was not so isolated. My friend Ron went out looking for firewood and fell down a mine shaft. I didn't go out that time.

You spend so much time with your work mates that you end up making great friends.

Anyway, after 9/11 it didn't seem like a good idea to be riding around with a shitload of guns and ammo and gun powder.

The party was over.

Breakfast at Willowick – December 17, 2012 2:14 P.M.

Willowick Golf Course is about a half-mile from where I live. I live in the 'hood, so by default, Willowick is in the 'hood. By the time you get to the second hole, a par three, you might as well be in Yosemite.

There's big, old trees, birds and squirrels running across the fairway…everything but bears and fish. There are no water hazards at the Wick either, just sand traps and trees. This is where we have the Annual Cinco de Mayo Tournament. 2013 will be the 25th year.

A few years ago, they built a nice clubhouse with a bar and restaurant. The food is good and the beer is cold. Prices are reasonable.

So when I started my first round of chemo in January of this year, my buddy from work, Steve Hallet, wanted to come visit me. He said he had a Christmas gift for me.

I had stopped working right before Christmas in 2011. My "Cancer-versary" is December 12, 2011. I'm borrowing cancer-versary from a fellow cancer warrior. Xeni Jardin who is kicking the crap out of breast cancer! I follow her on Twitter @xeni.

I started thinking of different places to go get some grub here in Santa Ana – there are so many. But then I started to think about my being on chemo and the "what ifs."

What if I felt sick?

What if I couldn't get to the bathroom?

What if I threw up right there in the restaurant?

What, what, what...

Then, I remembered about Willowick and that they served breakfast and lunch. It's close to the house, there's plenty of bathrooms and it's never too busy. Plus, there's plenty of parking.

Win, Win! Willowick it is!

I ordered an omelet and struggled to finish it but I did my best. Chemo is such an up and down experience and that day was a down day but I didn't want Steve to know. He probably did anyway.

His gift was a Kenny Powers shirt! Now, almost a year later, I'll be wearing the shirt Wednesday when I start chemo again.

We talked about work and stuff. It was a great visit and I really needed it. It got me out of the house.

The clubhouse at Willowick became and is still a favorite place to go eat. Steak and eggs for $6.99! And it's a real New York steak too. I've been there many times with Frank, Fran, Chris, my brothers, Janice, and even my mom.

What I'm really looking forward to is getting healthy so I can play a round of golf at the Wick!

It's a Wrap – December 18, 2012 4:59 P.M.

After my colostomy surgery I came home and the St. Joseph Home Health staff took over. Nurses would come to my house three times a week to help in my recovery and boy did I need help.

My surgeon, Dr. Anita Gregory, also made sure that one of the nurses would help me with my colostomy. That nurse was Keith and he's an expert with ostomies. While I was in the hospital two nurses showed me the basics of how to put on the colostomy bag. My sister Denise was there to help and also learn the procedure. I don't remember much but they were very nice.

When you take off the bag you use an adhesive remover to clean your skin around the stoma, then you use this skin prep (which is just an alcohol swab) to dry the area. After that you have to measure the stoma since it will still be shrinking down to its final form. That takes about a month.

So you measure and then cut out a hole in the part that sticks to your skin. It's called a skin barrier or a flange and that's the part that the bag is attached to. Now you can stick that to your skin then attach the bag and you're all ready to poop.

I had heard all about Keith in the hospital and was looking forward to meeting an expert. Besides the colostomy, I was a mess. I was draining from the front and the back. My surgery was a mother fucker!

I had sutures in my ass and staples from my belly button down to my pelvic area. I was constantly leaking so much that I finally asked my brother Kevin to go to Target and get me some Depends.

Washing my chonies[2] became a full-time job so I might as well just throw them away. I also had to add a feminine napkin to catch all the stuff coming out from behind.

In the hospital, I had two nurses emptying all my drains and urine Foley catheter, 24/7. But once I came home, it was all me, other than the three visits a week from Home Health.

I was getting stressed out about having to remember to empty this, change that, clean this…damn!

So, I finally meet Keith and we go to my room so he can do all the nurse stuff. Then he starts with the colostomy bag.

He pulls it off and cleans the area with a damp towel then dries it. He eyes my stoma and cuts out the hole on the skin barrier, slaps it on with the bag - slam bam thank you ma'am!

He tells me that I don't need all that skin prep and adhesive remover and that I have "good skin" so keep it simple.

Wow.

Was I impressed! I couldn't wait to tell Denise. Once my stoma shrank down to its permanent size, I was allowed to order precut skin barriers so I would no longer have to measure and cut out the hole.

Sweet.

Keith also told me to just eat healthy and that I should be fine.

When I was first told about having a colostomy I went to the internet and read all I could find about diet and it seemed very strict and limited. But, I follow the word of Keith and so far so good!

Since the first week of August until today, Keith and the other nurses from Home Health have been a huge part of my life and recovery. I had no idea that there was this whole other group of

---

2   Chicano slang for underwear.

nurses that just did house visits all day every day. I was even visited on Thanksgiving! Keith and Bernice and Nancy, thank you so much.

I shook Keith's hand today and thanked him. He wished me luck with my chemo.

The Beginning of the End – December 20, 2012 9:05 P.M.

Yesterday, I started six sessions of chemotherapy along with 12 sessions of Erbitux. The chemo will be every two weeks and the Erbitux every week. So let's see how it goes. So many things can happen…loss of hair, loss of weight, skin disorders, and diarrhea and on and on.

The first time I did chemo, I didn't lose my hair nor did I lose much weight. My appetite stayed half-way strong. I never threw up or suffered the craps. But I'm not taking anything for granted.

If I lose my hair, believe me it will grow back and I can stand to lose some weight, the way I eat….burp. This Erbitux is new for me and one of the side effects is a skin rash. The nurse said it's a good thing because then they know it's working.

Lucky me.

I could care less about all these side effects. I just want to get rid of this cancer and move on - back to a somewhat normal life! It's been a year now. I never imagined it going this long. Six months tops but you can never plan these things.

I felt like shit when I got home so I took some anti-nausea pills and then smoked some medical marijuana. In fact, I just stocked up on it the other day. I have an MM card that I got in February.

I go to this place where there's a "doctor" and I'm sitting there in this room where it's obvious I'm the only really sick person there. I mean, here I am carrying a chemo pump [3]and everyone else just looks stoned.

Anyway, I got my approval letter and was off to the nearest dispensary. It's a pretty cool place; jars and jars of weed with names that seemed were made up while on the weed in the jar. They also carry edibles such as cookies, brownies, Rice Krispy treats and candy with hash in it.

---

3   When chemotherapy is given through a central line or a PICC line, a pump can be attached to give a controlled amount of drugs very slowly into your bloodstream. Most pumps are "continuous pressure" pumps, which mean that they do not require a battery.

I tried them all.

I liked the brownies the best but what really got me stoned and partially paralyzed was the Hubby Bar. It's a chocolate candy divided into six pieces infused with hash.

All you need is one piece.

That's all I needed. I just stared at the TV. I couldn't move, not even to change the channel.

And I didn't feel the chemo…that's the bottom line.

The anti-nausea pills are good and all but the medical marijuana is so strong now that I highly recommend it if you ever have the unfortunate luck of getting cancer.

I've had this chemo pump for two days, so tomorrow I'll go and get unhooked. I'll repeat this five more times every two weeks and then, I hope I will be done.

It Was a Merry Christmas – December 25, 2012 10:33 P.M.

So many people put such high expectations on the holidays and then end up crying their asses off when things don't go the way they imagined. I like to keep my expectations low, very low.

At this point, Christmas is for kids; let them enjoy what's left of their childhood. They'll find out soon enough.

Tomorrow will be one week since my chemo and Erbitux treatments started. I already feel a little weak. My immune system has been compromised. That didn't take long.

Tomorrow I get another two-hour drip of Erbitux. Soon, I will have a rash on my skin and I can already feel the itching. Overall, my appetite is fine. For Christmas, I ate like there was no tomorrow; tamales, cookies, fudge, and the main course, prime rib with baked potato. Damn!

I was so happy to help with the tamales. My mom is getting up there and everyone else works so it's left upon my sister and she's getting tired of doing all the work. The recipe we use, is my grandmother's, from my mom's side.

They came here from Guanajuato, Mexico a long-long time ago. My mom is the last link to this recipe. All her brothers and sisters have died and none of our cousins even know the recipe, or care. So we made about ten pounds of meat, just enough to carry on the tradition - a boutique operation.

I videotaped as much as I could, especially when my mom made the chilé. She does everything from scratch. I helped Denise spread the masa on the hojas and then I passed out.

Hey, it's a start!

The final product was beautiful gems of stuffed maize. We don't shred the meat. I cut the pork meat into small bite size chunks that my mom simmers but doesn't fully cook. When Denise puts them together she puts an olive and some raisins in the tamale.

A friend, who is an expert in the history of Mexican food, said that putting an olive in the tamale was "very Chicano" of us. Ha! We only know what we know.

Some ancestor in Guanajuato put that olive in there, or maybe it was something my grandma picked up on the way to the U.S.

She was married at 15 and immediately set out for Los Estados Unidos and had her kids along the way, ending with my mom here in Stanton, California in 1925. My grandfather built their house in Stanton and it's still there.

In our little gifts of tamale you get some tender chunks of pork, a nice red sauce, some raisins and an olive.

Merry Christmas.

The Physical I Can't Control – December 30, 2012 4:30 P.M.

Right away, I realized that I would be subjected to numerous tests and treatments. When my primary care doctor gave me the bad news, it took all of ten seconds for me to ask him, "Now what do we do?"

When one is told that they have cancer the reactions do vary. Some people break down and cry. I would cry later.

Dr. Lin had already made two important appointments for me. The next day I was scheduled for a CT scan (computed axial tomography) and then on Wednesday I would meet with Dr. Anita Gregory, my surgeon. Things started to happen as fast as they could.

Consider the fact that the holiday was approaching and people were going on vacation. So on Monday, December 12, I found out the bad news.

I called work right away to tell them I wouldn't be in, for a while. On Tuesday, there was the CT scan and on Thursday, Dr. Gregory performed a colonoscopy. Wham, bam thank you ma'am!

The next week I had a PET Scan (Positron Emission Tomography) and then I met Dr. Ash, radiologist and Dr. Mahmood, oncologist; My Dream Team.

Other than the occasional flu bug I've never had to miss work for any length of time. Talking to my boss at work about the fact that I wouldn't be around for the two busiest weeks of the year, I was concerned about who would take my place.

All he said was, "Don't worry about it. Just get better."

As soon as he said those words, I felt like he lifted all the responsibility of my job and put it in another place. Somewhere, later (much later), I could go and retrieve this responsibility. But for now, my main job would be to take care of my health.

I can't thank Mark (my boss) enough for doing that. It was very simple but I needed to hear that.

So, I focused on everything that all my doctors were telling me. I organized every document. I became a student of cancer, of my health benefits and of state disability.

So many things were being thrown at me; medical terminology, tests, treatments. I had to become as mentally tough as I could. I had to constantly psyche myself up for whatever test they would throw at me.

I had a PICC line (peripherally inserted central catheter) inserted into my left arm. It's a port that they use for chemo drugs. I've never had one before but it was a fairly simple process. Still, the unknown can be scary.

I started saying Hail Marys over and over, as many as it would take to calm me down before the procedure. During my radiation treatment I must have said over a thousand Hail Marys.

I had heard that radiation was very simple and that it only took a few minutes for them to "zap" you and you were out of there. Easy breezy, my ass. Because of the nature of my cancer, I had a tumor that came out through the skin of my left buttock. Usually rectal/colon cancer will spread to the liver but not mine.

"Highly unusual" is what all three doctors would say when I initially met them. So my radiation treatments were longer and more intense than normal. They lasted about 12 to 15 minutes apiece.

Sometimes the computer would stop communicating to the machine (the machine that shoots out the laser beams) and it would stop working for about another 15 minutes.

So I would be laying there bare butt and exposed while they tried to re-boot the machine.

Hail Mary full of grace! became my mantra. I would be agitated and ask them, "Hello? Is this machine safe?"

I didn't feel comfortable at all with a machine shooting radiation up my ass that kept breaking down. After the sixth time of breaking down they reconfigured the sequence and it never broke down again.

Getting zapped in the ass was the easy part; the result of all that radiation was what I couldn't control – the physical.

By the end of the first week of radiation I didn't have any skin around my rectum…and I had to go for five more weeks of treatment, totaling 28 sessions in all. Plus, I carried a chemo pump, 24/7, the whole six weeks.

I can honestly say that I was mentally done by the sixth week. I was at the 24-mile mark of a 26-mile marathon and I didn't think I could finish.

I could no longer psyche myself up and going to the bathroom felt like lava was pouring out of my ass.

After the radiation treatment was done it took about three to four weeks before I got back to normal, meaning normal bowel movement without screaming or crying.

I thought: wow I made it.

What could possibly be worse than radiation..?

My surgery.

Another New Year but Who's Counting? – December 31, 2012 10:43 P.M.

I've had so many drunken New Year's celebrations; a sober one is now more common. In fact, at this point in my life I think I've had more of these quiet evenings.

Tonight is what they call amateur night. It's when all those rookies go out and get sloshed, get DUI's or get into an accident. Pretty sad. Usually, I have to work New Year's Day.

One New Years that stands out for me was when I was married. My ex-wife's grandmother lived in Pasadena, off of Orange Grove, where the Rose Parade starts, less than a block away from the parade.

The granddaddy of them all!

I had never been. Even after being married for a while I'd still rather work and get the triple time rather than party. I'd show up later for dinner but had never experienced the whole New-Years-Eve-on-the-parade-route, overnight thing.

My wife's grandmother, Colleen or Cokie, contracted pancreatic cancer. Pancreatic cancer is probably the one cancer that you just can't beat. She seemed to be doing well though.

We were there for Thanksgiving dinner and Cokie personally asked me to attend the New Year's festivities. How could I refuse?

This tradition had been going on for years and years. The family had it down to a science. They still had to go out and save spots on the street but it was all organized with the neighbors. From the food to the hot cocoa to the morning sweets, everything was great. It was definitely not their first time at the rodeo.

We would go hang out and save the seats then someone would take our place while we went inside to warm up. Why hadn't I joined this party before?

All of Cokie's family was there; she had four sons plus grandkids, and family from Arizona. It was a full and festive house. Cokie never did leave the house that day, she watched the parade on TV instead. She had plenty of friends and family to entertain.

I had a great time for my first Rose Parade experience with all the comforts of home.

Everyone left as the day went on. All except the family from Arizona. They stayed a few extra days

As soon as they left, Cokie went to bed but before she fell asleep she called her son, Mick. All she said was, "Mick…"

That was it.

Cokie knew she only had so much time left. She made sure all her family was there, including me, one last time. One last New Year's.

All the kids and all the adults acting like kids, having the time of their life. She sat there watching everyone, making sure we were warm enough, had enough to eat. And when the last guest left, when the last hugs and good-byes were said, Cokie passed on.

An amazing woman.

To hold on like that, not letting on how bad she was suffering… from the moment she asked me to attend she knew her time was near. I'm glad everyone was there one last time.

It was a very special New Year's.

Chemo Session #2 – January 1, 2013 10:03 P.M.

Tomorrow will be my second of six chemo sessions and third session of Erbitux. The first session went well; I didn't realize how hard the chemo had hit me last Friday.

I thought I was tired but after four hours of resting, I came to the conclusion that I was being "chemotized." What's really starting to affect me is the Erbitux. It's the additional drug that will keep oxygen from the cancer and help kill it. Suffocate it. Fuck it.

The side effect is an acne-like rash. Now, in my teens, I had pimples but never an acne problem. Nurse Mindy told me that it makes them happy to see the rash because that's how they know the Erbitux is working.

Well Mindy…I hope you're happy!

All around my nose are these little whitehead-like pimples but they're not pimples. They bleed.

I woke up yesterday with dried scabs around my nose. I showered and used the medicated soap they gave me; an Aveeno product. I patted dry my face, but I still popped a few of these so called pimples and they started to bleed.

So tomorrow, I will be looking for some kind of relief .I understand it's part of the deal; kill cancer, get some bloody acne. So I'm good with it and the nurses did tell me that they can prescribe me something if it got out of hand, or even stop the treatment if it got that bad.

I'm not complaining. No way, José.

St. Joseph Hospital is where I get all my treatments and where I had my surgery. It's one of the best hospitals in Orange County. They also have the Children's Hospital of Orange County. It's right across the street from the Cancer Center.

And that's why I don't complain.

Through my previous chemo and radiation treatments there were no complaints. Not me. Because in that CHOC hospital are kids – little kids, babies going through Hell. Chemo Hell, radiation Hell…they're my inspiration. That they can still smile is beyond my comprehension.

I've been very fortunate to have such great support from friends and family. I can physically feel all the positive thoughts and prayers.

Really.

It's overwhelming and I take all that love and good karma and send it over to CHOC. This is how I thank you.

Just in case there is a child over there that's not as lucky as I am to have the support of great friends and family, then take my overflow. Please. Ease that pain.

I know it hurts.

Two Down, Four to Go – January 4, 2013 7:14 P.M.

Or so I thought. Today, I went in to have the chemo pump removed. 48-hours of continuous toxic liquid pumping into my body.

I thanked the nurse. See you next week! Two down, four to go!

"I'm not too sure about that, Robert. Let me check. It looks like you're booked until April. Twelve chemo sessions," she said.

I thought she was joking so I smiled and then she smiled but it was no joke - just the hard truth.

I was originally told that all I needed was six sessions of chemo plus 12 sessions of the Erbitux. And that's what I was mentally prepared for. Now, I was looking at six more sessions of chemo plus more Erbitux.

The nurse, Christine, said that I will be evaluated again after the first six sessions and that I might not need the other six but they want me to give the heads up to my insurance just in case.

They also had to write a letter to my job to let them know how much longer I'll be out.

But still I need to know if my prognosis has changed…I'm always the last to know! It's not bad news, just unexpected. I'll survive. No doubt.

Deep breaths, Robert. Deep breaths.

Where the Fuck Have I Been? – January 8, 2013 4:55 P.M.

Let's see, the last time I wrote here was on Friday. That seems like a month ago. The chemo seems to really be knocking me out. Of course, it won't let me sleep.

Wednesday night: no sleep.

Thursday night: no sleep.

Friday night: nada sleep.

But on Sunday, I slept all day. And I won't really call it "sleep" per se; it's more like being knocked out with a sledgehammer. I tried to watch football but there was just no way. Oh well.

Monday was better. I made dinner; fresh pico de gallo with rice and beans, grilled some chicken. Good stuff. I watched Notre Dame get their ass kicked.

I'm just trying to go with whatever energy level I have for that day. If I can accomplish any chores then great but if chemo knocks me out then what can I do but sleep it off?

Tomorrow I go in for more Erbitux. That's a two-hour drip and the side effect is the skin rash which I'm taking antibiotics for.

My Sons of Anarchy marathon is almost over. Not bad. I think it's funny that they spend more time in the hospital than I ever did.

My surgery kept me in the hospital for eight days. I was a little shocked when they sent me home. I was a complete mess.

I guess they needed the bed.

When Your Surgeon Tells You You Need a Colostomy – January 10, 2013 4:33 P.M.

I met all three doctors and came away very impressed. I began chemo in January of 2012 for three months and then without skipping a beat I went right into radiation while hooked up to a chemo pump 24/7.

This lasted for six weeks.

And then they finally let me rest. My insides were fried. But after three to four weeks, things are almost back to normal. The skin around my rectum is healed; in fact it's brand new.

Woo hoo! I can poop without screaming.

Now it's time to meet with Dr. Gregory, my surgeon.

I had a basic idea of the game plan from day one; chemo, radiation, surgery, recovery and then back to work. And I thought all this would happen in about six months. Well, I was wrong.

My meeting with Dr. Gregory didn't happen until late May so the soonest we could do surgery was mid-June. I had to get an extension from work and my state disability. Dr. Gregory estimated my return to work would be in September.

I go into her office and we sit down and the first thing she tells me is that I need to have a permanent colostomy.

Boom.

She said that I would be able to do everything that I used to do; work, swim, sex, eat…except I would be pooping in a bag that would be attached to the front left side of my abdomen - a stoma.

My rectum and sphincter muscle would be completely removed.

Gone.

In a bucket.

The operation would take about four and half hours. It would be a robotic surgery; snip-snip, through two small incisions and then everything would be pulled out through my rectum which would then be sewed up for eternity.

Really?

I felt like turning around to make sure it was me she was talking to. I just kept nodding my head as if I knew all along this was going to happen. But I didn't have a clue that this was my only option…

I stayed calm and got up and said: Okay.

I mumbled something about scheduling it as soon as possible, but the whole time I'm already formulating a letter in my head with a million questions.

I went home in a daze and researched everything I could about colostomies and sphincter and rectal cancer. And I wrote Dr. Gregory a letter telling her that while I wasn't exactly looking for a second opinion, I did need a whole lot of information so that I could get on board with this colostomy which would change my life forever.

Dr. Gregory answered each of my questions.

I asked her why did I have to go through all that chemo and radiation if we were going to pull the whole thing out anyway? Why not just do the colostomy first then treat what cancer was left with chemo or radiation?

That probably would have been easier on me but apparently over many years they have found that by doing chemo and radiation first, the cancer has a far less chance of reoccurring.

I told her that since my sphincter was working great couldn't we just cut out the tumor? What would be my chances of survival?

Well, it turns out that the tumor had compromised my sphincter so it was a textbook case to pull it all out. To do that would give me a 95-percent chance of survival.

No one had ever not pulled out the rectum and sphincter and she could only guess that my survival rate would be 50-percent at best if I did not go through with it.

It was everything that I needed to hear.

The next week she even presented my case to the tumor board at

St. Joseph which is made up of about 20 cancer surgeons, including my radiologist and oncologist. They all agreed that I had to have the colostomy.

Fine.

One more question.

When I was first diagnosed, I took about 10 seconds to think about the fact that I was just told I had cancer, then I asked so what do we do now?

I never asked what stage cancer I had.

I didn't feel that it was all that important…

All I wanted to do was to get rid of the cancer, regardless of the stage. Throughout my treatment I was asked by various friends what stage I was in and I didn't have the answer.

So I finally asked Dr. Gregory and she said I was stage three but with the size and placement of the tumor I was now stage four.

Wow.

No Popcorn?! WTF – January 13, 2013 5:56 P.M.

After Dr. Gregory answered all my questions I would say I was about 80-percent on board with the whole colostomy thing. And it was a strong 80-percent.

Of course there were still some questions that could only be answered after I have surgery. How will the colostomy affect me at work?

I really love my job and can't wait to get back to work but will I be able to do my job? It will be interesting but I don't see having a colostomy interfering with how I work. Accidents do happen but I will be prepared for those.

Hey, shit happens.

My internet research covered everything I could think of, especially how your diet affects your colostomy and vice versa. There's so much information on what you can eat and what you can't eat.

How to eat.

Chewing is even more important than ever!

When they remove your rectum and your sphincter you're going to need some help. You want things to move along as smoothly as possible. So there's this list of foods to avoid – foods that might hinder the movement of your now diverted digestive system. And the one food that jumped out from my laptop screen was POPCORN.

I was no longer allowed to eat popcorn?

I guess it doesn't digest easily. BUT I LOVE POPCORN. There, I said it. Popcorn is THE reason I go to the movies. I even have my own personal bucket.

The theatre I go to sells this medium sized container for $6 then after that the refills are $3. Same for the soda. It's a great deal.

I loved popcorn...

What was really keeping me from getting to be 100-percent behind the colostomy was fear. I had this tremendous fear that the colostomy would change me as a person. I was afraid that I would wake up after the surgery and look at the colostomy bag and just be very angry, very bitter and not be able to get over the fact that for the rest of my life I would have to poop in a bag.

Remember, wiping your ass is a privilege, not a right.

I was just scared to death. Like a prisoner on death row I was waiting for the last minute reprieve - the call from the Governor.

"Stop! Stop the colostomy!"

But it never came.

In pre-op as I was waiting with my family. They sent in a nurse to measure the exact spot for the stoma. Apparently she's an expert at this. She was very nice and it only took a few minutes but I was a marked man.

Shit.

This was really going to happen.

Getting mentally prepared for this surgery was so hard. I thought because of all my questions, that they might get me some kind of help. A therapist...the mental kind.

And I asked about support groups, which they have but I was really looking for someone like me, age-wise, but there wasn't anyone else like me that was getting a colostomy. But I had to talk to someone.

I needed to talk to someone.

I'm a firm believer in old sayings. Specifically, "everything happens for a reason." And for some reason, I met a friend through work, a salesperson, a very nice girl named Maria Antonia Villalobos.

We talk. We're friends and for a week she listened to all my fears and thoughts. She said all the right things, she didn't judge or really give any major opinion. But by the end of three or four nights of conversation I was over my fear.

I had accepted my fate.

I would not let the colostomy or cancer change me or my life. I vowed to take charge and become an expert in everything about colostomies.

Fuck you, Cancer!

This is My life.

Chemo Session #3 – January 17, 2013 5:09 P.M.

All I can say is so far so good. As I become more saturated with the chemo solution then I will probably feel worse but for now my appetite is good. I keep everything down.

The one thing that is kicking my ass is the 25ml of Benadryl they give me every week to start my treatment. It knocks me OUT. And it is now affecting the way I sleep at night, or I should say the way I'm not sleeping at night.

I fell asleep at 8 a.m. this morning only to wake back up at 9 a.m. I had a 9:40 appointment with my primary Doctor. Other than the lack of sleep, I can't complain.

I'm killing cancer right now.

Last year was the first time in over twenty years that I didn't make our annual Super Bowl trip to Vegas. My brothers and friends and a whole bunch of people we don't know have been making this a fun event. But I was doing chemo and didn't want to be a burden on my brothers.

This year I decided I would go. I realized my mom would be all alone but she is fine and does enjoy her alone time. So I will be going to Vegas this weekend! Woo hoo! Fuck you, Cancer! Asshole!

I'll be fine. It should be a lot of fun watching the AFC and NFC championship games. Making my little bets…the over? The under? Parlay the final score to the first half over/under? Yeah, just like Super Bowl Sunday. Then, after the games, the sports books will post the odds for the super Bowl and I can make my bets for that game. Winner!

I've been battling this damn cancer for over a year and I need a little respite from all this that has become my life. And rightly so. I've completely devoted all my daily effort to do whatever my doctors want or need me to do. I've been a model patient and I need to get away, even if just for a few days.

I'll be staying in the Downtown Las Vegas area at the El Cortez Hotel. Old School. It's cheap and clean. Right across the street is Mamacita's, and they have the best Mexi-Cuban food. They will do your dish either Mexi style or Cuban style. Great breakfast. Awesome Cuban sandwich and very affordable.

So I better rest up! :)

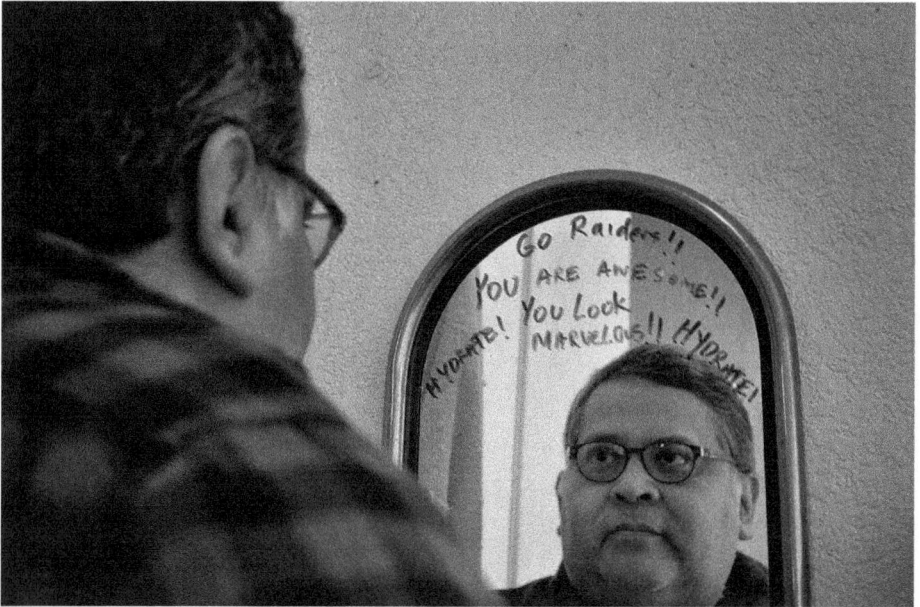

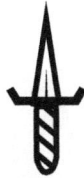

Part II: The Devil's Dagger

Four Years Ago – January 18, 2013 11:22 P.M.

I was getting ready to fly out to witness the inauguration of President Obama, all thanks to Janice Briones, my longtime friend and neighbor. Right after Obama was elected Janice made hotel reservations for the inauguration.

Back then, Janice would travel for business so she was able to use her frequent-flyer miles. She told me she would be staying at the Hilton in Crystal City by the airport but as the day grew closer Janice found out she had to fly out to Guam for business that weekend so she wouldn't be able to attend the inauguration.

So Janice called me and asked if I would like the room so it wouldn't go to waste.

Hmmm…let me think about this…Hell yeah!

I asked my sister, Denise, if she'd like to go(she lives in Seattle) and was the only other person like me that could get the time off – by plane, train and bus – just go!

Flying into D.C. was well over $600 and going up every time I clicked a website. The algorithms were not in my favor. We decided to fly into New York City and take a $20 bus ride to D.C. which was still way cheaper than $600.

Denise flew into Newark and I flew into JFK and we met at Penn Station. This was the beginning of an epic adventure. Planning and coordinating a trip like this was right up my alley. I love doing this kind of stuff.

Denise is a world class traveler. Once we got to D.C. she had the Metro maps ready and she did some research into the places to eat around our hotel area. She rocks, my sister.

We arrived at the hotel while a huge concert was going on at the National Mall. We watched the end of it on TV then decided to go to the Mall and find our route for the big day.

Crystal City is very close and convenient to the Mall and I'm sure Janice had that all figured out. The Metro got us there in minutes and right away you could feel the excitement in the air.

We did our walk about and headed back to find a place to eat and watch an NFL playoff game. I remember the Ravens were playing. Denise had a few places in mind but they were packed. We found a place that wasn't so busy – Ted's Montana Grill. We sat at the bar and they had the game on.

At Ted's you can have your steak or burger either bison or choice beef. I had the bison burger and Denise had chicken under a brick. Both were bomb dot com.

We went back the next night and in fact, we ate there all three nights. Now, I know better and traveling to different cities means eating at a different place every night but Ted's was that good and it was right by our hotel. We also spotted a Chipotle and bought burritos for the inauguration – have burrito will travel.

The one touristy thing that we did was visit the Holocaust Museum and it was unbelievable.

I thought I knew a lot about the Holocaust. I was wrong. If you ever get the chance, go but be warned, it's devastating.

Inauguration morning; we bundle up, burritos ready. The Metro is packed like sardines. A girl faints but doesn't fall down because it's so packed.

Estimates of up to a million people are expected to attend this event. And it is cold.

The burritos turned to popsicles but everything went very well. There were plenty of porta-potties. I had downloaded this guide: Where to Pee in D.C., before I left home. I never had to use it but I was prepared.

Security, of course, was going to be huge; no taxis or buses and they closed all the Metro entrances except for one. We knew this beforehand and decided that if we had to we would walk back to Crystal City. And we did.

After spending all morning and afternoon at the Mall we realized that walking back made more sense than trying to get on the Metro, and we weren't the only ones. We made it back to the hotel in one piece, rested and then went back to Ted's for some steaks. I had the rib eye, Denise had filet mignon.

We had just witnessed History.

I splurged on Amtrak tickets to get out of D.C. No bus because I was afraid we might get stuck in a massive traffic jam and miss our planes.

We got back to New York and Denise decided to visit Rockefeller Center before she flew out. I declined.

I was tired, but not too tired to enjoy a couple slices of

N.Y. pizza.

The Big Day – January 21, 2013 10:21 P.M.

My surgery was scheduled for Thursday, July 26. It should have been in June, but I went through that whole freak out period and Dr. Gregory submitted my case to the tumor board. Then Dr. Gregory had a vacation coming up, so July 26 it was.

Ready or not.

But I was ready.

Let's do this!

Please.

So…things didn't go exactly as planned. A four and a half hour surgery turned into an eight hour ordeal. Of course I had no idea what had happened. When I woke up everyone started to fill me in.

It was great to see my family and friends. They hung in there and waited and waited for the surgery to finish. The robotic method didn't work out so I was split open. Right away, I knew my recovery was going to be longer and more complicated.

Dr. Gregory said my tumor was practically embedded into my pelvis. I call my tumor the "Devil's Dagger." Satan himself, punched a 13-centimeter long chunk of cancer into my butt and said, "Good luck with that!"

Whatever.

Dick.

This is my first surgery ever. I've never had to stay in a hospital for anything. Ever! St. Joseph is a great hospital for a first timer. Dr. Gregory was there every morning. Of course, I was being closely monitored; nurses coming in to empty this, check that. I had staples from my belly button all the way down to my pelvic area, a brand new colostomy, and my backside had also been opened up. I had stuff coming out of everywhere.

I was a mess and in pain. The pain...the Pain!

The first few days are a total blur; I just kept pushing that button that made the pain go away. After a few days in recovery I got a regular room to myself. Nice.

Right away, they want you to get up and walk around.

Really.

Just to the door and back, Robert...

Ok, I can do that. The food was pretty good – made to order. I was a mess but I was doing OK...until they took off the Foley catheter that is.

They need to know if you can pee on your own. They use the word void. So they remove the catheter and give me four hours to void.

If you can't void we have to put the catheter back on.

Oh, no.

Of course I couldn't void. So there goes the Foley and I fill a bag up right away.

One more try.

What?

The nurse removes the catheter again and says: good luck.

Are you kidding?

If I couldn't go earlier what would make them think I could void now?

And I didn't. So they put the catheter back in.

Right now I will tell you that I lost count how many times I had to have the Foley put on and off.

Torture. Pure torture.

Something was wrong, so Dr. Gregory brought in urologist, Dr. Vorouzi. He started me on Flomax. This relationship would last about five months.

After eight days I was released from the hospital, even though I felt I could have stayed at least another week. I would have St. Joseph Home Health nurses coming over to my house three times a week to help me.

I also had an appointment with Dr. Vorouzi the next week and hopefully, I would be able to void on my own and get rid of this catheter.

Torture. Pure torture…

My Time in the Hospital was Such a Blur – January 24, 2013 5:38 P.M.

In the beginning….I was seriously hallucinating during my stay in the hospital. It must have been all the meds and pain stuff I was getting. I woke up one night, looked around, found my phone and called my compadre.

"Where are you? Where's everybody at? I need to get out of here!" It was along those lines. I don't really remember.

You're not allowed to eat the day before surgery, or the day of surgery. My third day in the hospital, when I was still on a liquid diet, I started to complain. That made it five days without solid food and I was Hungry!

"NURSE! NURSE! Oh, it's 2 a.m., Can I get some real food?"

"No. Your doctor still has you on a liquid diet; Jell-O, tea."

"But I'm starving! Can I get a peanut butter sandwich? Please? Half a peanut butter sandwich?

"NO."

"So can you call my doctor and tell her that I'm very hungry for some food that isn't Jell-O?"

"No! It's 2 a.m.!"

"I don't care!"

I wasn't getting anywhere. She's responsible for me...she put me here...I'm a grown man!

They gave me a couple of pain meds and I knocked out. But by the next day I was on a solid food diet. Three meals a day, made to order according to the diet I was on. Not bad.

I was almost ready to go across the street to Carl's Jr. (it's open 24 hours) just for a bite of a burger...anything! Five days without solid food, that's crazy!

I'm Catholic, so are my family and most of my friends. I'm not the best Catholic, but I do my best. My Mom and brothers and sister visited me every day, as did my friends. One day, I was there with my mom and a volunteer walked in and offered to give us Communion.

Well, I haven't been to confession since...but he said it was OK, some kind of dispensation blah, blah, blah, in the name of the Father, Son, and Holy Ghost. Wow. That was cool, receiving Communion with my Mom. She was very happy. It became a daily event and very spiritual.

I really appreciated the opportunity to do that with my Mom. I think we both needed it. It couldn't hurt.

Just by pushing a button you can get a dose of pain medicine. As soon as the light goes back on you can push the button again for another dose. Very Pavlovian. Then, after so many days of pain med Nirvana, they switch you over to a solid pill. No more instant happy.

They gave me the equivalent of 2,500mg Vicodin and I immediately passed out. I was still on an empty stomach at this time, so it hit me hard. The nurse on duty made note of this and my next dose was Tylenol 3 with codeine. Huh?

"What happened to the Vicodin?"

"It was too strong for you."

"I was on an empty stomach, of course I passed out. These Tylenol 3 don't do the trick. I'm in a lot of pain here...

Nothing.

I told my Doctor.

Nothing.

Great.

They release me from the hospital.

Go home.

Good luck.

Some very nice older volunteers take you in a wheelchair down to the area where we waited for my brother to bring his car around, and waited, and waited, I needed to stand up. Sitting down was still very painful.

It had only been eight days since my surgery and all I was getting was Tylenol 3 with codeine. I tried to stand up but the volunteer pushed me back into the wheelchair.

Ouch!

That hurt.

Finally, Jeff pulled up.

I could barely get in the car fast enough. My butt was killing me. We live about 10-minutes from St. Joseph. Nice. I went directly to my room.

I had a big bottle of Vicodin left over from my radiation treatment. 750 mg. I took one every four hours.

The pain went bye-bye.

Recovering From Surgery is a Full-Time Job – January 26, 2013 4:16 P.M.

I didn't realize this. In the hospital I had two full-time nurses, 24/7. They were always doing something to me; emptying this, filling that, take your pills, check your blood pressure, all day and all night. I get home and of course my family is there to help me and three times a week a nurse comes over. The Home Health nurses are very nice but when they're not there I'm pretty much on my own to do all the stuff they were doing inside the hospital.

I was draining from the front, but Dr. Gregory removed the drain and the receptacle that all the fluid was going into. The back was a mess too – more fluid draining. Yuck.

The day after I came home I was in the kitchen getting a snack, a fruit cup, and all this ugly liquid came out my front. What a mess. I had no warning, I did have gauze over my incision but damn.

This became so frequent that we just put newspapers on the floor in the bathroom to help catch all this messy stuff.

After about a week, I asked my brother Kevin to go to Target and get me some Depends. Yep, Depends. It was becoming a full time job to keep my underwear dry and clean so I said let's go with the Depends and just throw them away. I would have to wear them for at least 2 months but it was the way to go.

I was pretty much in bed all the time. Sitting was still very painful and would be, for a while. I needed help for everything. I had the Foley catheter and that was a constant pain in the wiener. I would try my best not to move or make any moves that would irritate the damn thing but it would still hurt. I didn't have any appointments for the first two weeks but after that, I would have to get myself ready to leave the house, where I felt safe, and start with the follow ups.

Besides the Depends, I was also wearing a feminine napkin to help with everything coming out my rectal area. I would probably change it three to four times a day. On the off days, when the nurse wouldn't be there, I would have to change my front bandages. That was easy but messy.

I do regret not taking a picture of all my staples while they were still in. The first time I saw the staples I was shocked. But it would have made an awesome picture…this is what my cancer looks like…staples from my belly button down to my pelvic area and my colostomy right next to it.

No CGI.

This was the real deal.

My first follow up was with Dr. Vorouzi, the urologist. That didn't go well. He was on vacation but he told me that his partner would know what to do. This visit would take place about three weeks after my surgery.

I still had the Foley catheter. They were to do a 'fill and void.' That's where they fill my bladder with saline and then take off the catheter and see if I can void on my own.

Well his partner didn't want to take off the catheter; he said it was too soon. He didn't even know me. I said no. Take it off.

So they took it off and I was sent home to see if I would void on my own. If nothing happened in five hours I would have to come back to have the catheter put back on.

I was 100% sure I would be able to go.

I drank water and juice and more water but nothing happened. By 4 p.m. I was back in the doctor's office where they put the Foley back on and I filled the bag right away. My bladder was still not ready. I was so bummed.

Before my surgery, I had gotten myself mentally prepared for three main things. Number one, was to make sure that after surgery, I would do everything I could to become an expert in handling my colostomy. I would be the best.

Number two, was to do everything to help my recovery; eat well, listen to my doctors, think positive.

And the third thing was to prepare myself in case I needed more chemo. I knew that would be a possibility even after surgery but if I needed more chemo, then I was all psyched up to do it.

What I wasn't prepared for was wearing this Foley catheter for so long. I guess my bladder got beat up pretty bad during surgery and needed time to recover. All I knew was that before my surgery, I could pee with the best of them, so I knew it was just a matter of time before I could go on my own. But this was taking too long.

Like I said before, I lost count how many times the catheter was taken off and put back on, and I bet you've lost count too.

Fuck the Bulls – January 30, 2013 10:13 P.M.

At this point in my life running with the bulls would be boring.

Chemo Session #4 – January 31, 2013 3:13 P.M.

Whew. Yesterday was my fourth session. And of course I didn't get much sleep last night. None – to be exact. I did eventually fall asleep this morning for a few hours.

So many ounces of toxic chemicals infused into me over a five hour period. Yuck. But I welcome this poison into my body. Do your thing Erbitux. Fuck that cancer, Camptosar (generically known as Irinotecan, which is used together with other medicines to treat cancer of the colon or rectum).

All my other vitals are doing well. I am anemic, not borderline, but not in need of a blood transfusion just yet. I've had two blood transfusions over the last year. The nurses will first give me a Procrit shot which usually does the trick.

I do not notice any difference in how I feel; whether I'm so anemic that I need the transfusion, (which is usually two pints of blood) or after the transfusion, I feel energized. I'm good.

During my next chemo session I will see my oncologist. I have some questions for him. I'm wondering when I will have a PET scan. I'm curious to see where the cancer is (or isn't) and whether I will need six sessions or twelve.

I gots to know.

I gots bills.

I gots to get back to work.

Yeah, work.

It's been over a year since I've been to work. Wow. I seriously thought this would all take about six months, tops. Nope. Not even close. But you can't really predict these things and all that could happen along that way.

It's been quite a journey.

My heartfelt thanks to everyone for your thoughts and prayers, your jokes, your chismes[4], the time you take to talk, text, Facebook, Twitter and Instagram. Very powerful.

At times I'm overwhelmed and that's a great thing.

---

4   Gossip.

Super Bowl Sunday in Vegas – February 2, 2013 11:13 A.M.

I'm baaaack. I was here two weeks ago as planned and now I'm here this weekend, not as planned. Usually my two brothers and I come to Las Vegas for the Super Bowl but I decided to come two weeks ago and watch the NFC and AFC championship games.

Then I would stay with my mom and watch the Super Bowl with her. Party time. But Jeff couldn't get the time off so I took one for the team and came with my other brother Killer Kevin.

Not having any luck at all but I'm having a great time and eating some good food. The prime rib last night at the El Cortez was tasty, tender and very affordable.

I'm pulling for the Ravens. I took the under in the first half, took the Lakers and the Clippers too.

I hope I win something…

Dump – February 5, 2013 2:00 P.M.

Sometimes I wish I could just sit down on the porcelain throne and take a dump, read the paper or browse through a magazine. It's the simple pleasure of life I miss.

Recovering From Surgery Continues – February 7, 2013 6:11 P.M.

My surgery was July 26, 2012 and I was in the hospital for eight days. When I came home a heat wave was just about to start up. I live in a house without an air conditioner but that never bothered me because I was always at work. And I happen to work in a constant 50 to 55-degree meat cooler – everyday, for the last 30-years.

Heat waves were not something my body was ready for. So I'm basically bed ridden the first month that I'm home and now I'm baking in my room, seriously. In the hospital the temp is controlled to prevent bacteria from growing. That's why it's usually so cold in there.

So now I really need to find an air conditioner but so is everyone else in Southern California. I call every Home Depot around. I'm on the internet searching. All sold out. Fuck. This is not good.

I'm trying to heal my wounds and trying to digest food with a colostomy here…I have a fan but come on, it's just fanning the hot air.

I tell my compadre Francisco about my search for an air conditioner and he takes it upon himself to go out and find one for me. He and comadre[5] Patty drive to every Home Depot and Lowes in Tustin and Santa Ana, they even went to Costco, but no luck.

Damn.

Then my friend Chris says his parents have one that they're not using, so Fran goes and picks it up, but it's missing a part, so now he enlists his brother George to "Mickey Mouse" it, and it works!

But not really – it won't get cold. I don't know why, but it won't.

Then Frank Martinez remembers that his parents also have a standalone air conditioner that they're not using, and it works! Really! It works and my room is at a constant 75-degrees.

Whew.

Let the healing begin.

Awesome friends.

My first visit with Dr. Norouzi didn't go so well and I'm to see him in a week. One more week with the catheter but I know for sure it will be gone the next time. My appointment is for Thursday the 16th of August.

I get into a habit of waking up around 1 a.m. to check the Foley bag and to empty it so it's not so full in the morning. It seems to fill up quite a bit when I fall asleep.

Tuesday the 14th I wake up and notice that the bag is empty, no urine. But when I move to get up I can feel my bladder is full. I need to go.

So I call the Home Health nurse, and by this time I have boxes of medical supplies everywhere. She tells me to find the box with the extra Foley supplies and to look for a huge plastic syringe.

She's going to talk me through on how to unblock my catheter so I

5   Sort of like saying "dude" but for a female. Compadre is the masculine version.

can void.

OK.

So here it is almost 2 a.m. and I cannot find this huge plastic syringe or the bottle of saline.

Sorry…It's just not in the box.

So now she has to send out a nurse in the middle of the night to unblock the catheter, and I have to pee…bad!

The nurse lives in Aliso Viejo so it's going to take her at least 35 to 45-minutes to get to my house. I'm doing ok but please hurry.

So she arrives, very nice lady, and she has the huge plastic syringe and tries not once but three times to unblock the catheter, no go.

She has to remove the catheter and put a new one on. As soon as she does the bag fills up, relief finally.

Thank you!

Two nights later on Thursday I wake up around 4 a.m. and the bag is empty.

Not again!

This time I really have to go but before I call the nurse I try myself to unblock the catheter. No luck, it's blocked.

Fuck.

Fuck…fuck!

I call the nurse and wait the 45-minutes but this time I am freaking out. I feel like I'm going to explode. Kevin wakes up and talks to me, tries to calm me down. I'm praying and trying to relax.

¡Ay, Dios mio!

The nurse shows up and she has to try to unblock the catheter but nope, she has to remove the catheter and put on a new one. Again!

Unbelievable.

I fill the bag up but I'm shaking and my blood pressure is through the roof. She doesn't understand how the catheter could block twice within two days.

Well, believe it.

And she shows me how to remove the catheter this time in case it happens again. My appointment with Dr. Norouzi is for later that day…

I show up at Dr. Norouzi's and fill him in on my adventures. He's going to do a fill and void and it goes well. They fill my bladder and as soon as they remove the catheter I void. I make arrangements with Home Health, in case this doesn't work out, so that they have a nurse on duty to come out and put a catheter on.

My appointment should have been for the morning but it was made for 4 p.m. I go home without a catheter. Yay! Freedom!

I'm drinking water and some cranberry juice. Home Health told me to call by 9 p.m. if I can't void on my own. Around 7 p.m. I have to go but just barely – just a trickle. And by 9 p.m. nothing.

So I call the nurse and she tells me to relax and give it some more time. Finally at 11:30 p.m. I have to go and I void big time, just like the old days.

Ha ha.

But I make a mess.

Bad aim I guess, I don't know, but there's some pee on the floor.

I clean up my mess and go to bed, very happy. At 1:30 a.m. I have to go again…and again I make a mess.

What the heck?

Is pee coming out of my butt too?

I clean up and go back to bed but I think that next time I will sit down and pee just in case pee is coming out of my butt.

4:30 a.m. I have to go and sort of sit down, but I want to see if I'm peeing from my butt. I look down and start to pee and I see nothing but blood coming out of my rectum area.

Holy fuck.

A lot of blood.

I stand up and finish peeing then clean up this bloody mess. I go back to bed to think about my options. What the hell just happened?! Should I go to emergency? It's almost 5 a.m. so I decide to call Dr. Gregory; her answering service puts me through after I explain what just happened.

Dr. Gregory tells me not to go the emergency room; she will call Dr. Norouzi, so he will be calling me, and so I wait. Around 8 a.m., his nurse tells me to come on in as soon as I can. I wake Kevin up and we go in to Dr. Norouzi's office.

Dr. Norouzi asks me a series of questions and decides that he needs to have me do a CT scan with a contrast liquid so he can see where the urine is coming out. I have to wait until about 11 a.m. to get this done.

They put on a catheter and fill my bladder with the contrast liquid and put me in the CT machine. Of course this is no picnic of a test.

I'm having flashbacks of Tuesday and Thursday, they have to put in so many CC's of the liquid in my bladder in order for the test to work. Finally the test is over. I go home and wait for the phone call for the results.

About 3 p.m. they call me and tell me to get over to Dr. Norouzi's office so he can go over the test results. I drive myself over there – the first time since my surgery that I have driven.

All things considered I'm doing ok. I pray constantly; the Hail Marys are my mantra. I sit down with Dr. Norouzi and it's bad news.

Probably the worst news since Dr. Gregory tells me I have to have a colostomy.

I have a fistula in my urethra: a small tear in the tube that leads from my bladder to my penis.

Dr. Norouzi tells me that these take a long time to heal…if it heals.

If?

"What do you mean 'if'?"

"Well, you have had a lot of radiation treatment in that area and that makes it hard for that area to heal. There are doctors which specialize in fixing these tears but you are a long way from that. You still have to deal with your cancer."

And then Dr. Gregory tells me that I had it pretty bad.

Wow.

I am reeling.

If it heals?

That's not right…I can heal. I'm a healer. Big time.

So for now Dr. Norouzi decides to slap on another Foley catheter. Are we keeping count still? But this one has a bigger gauge to avoid any more blockages.

Besides urine I'm passing a lot of mucus and weird debris which is causing the blockage. He says he'll see me in two weeks and see where we go from there.

Now I have to get into my truck and drive home.

Fuck me, again.

#FuckCancer

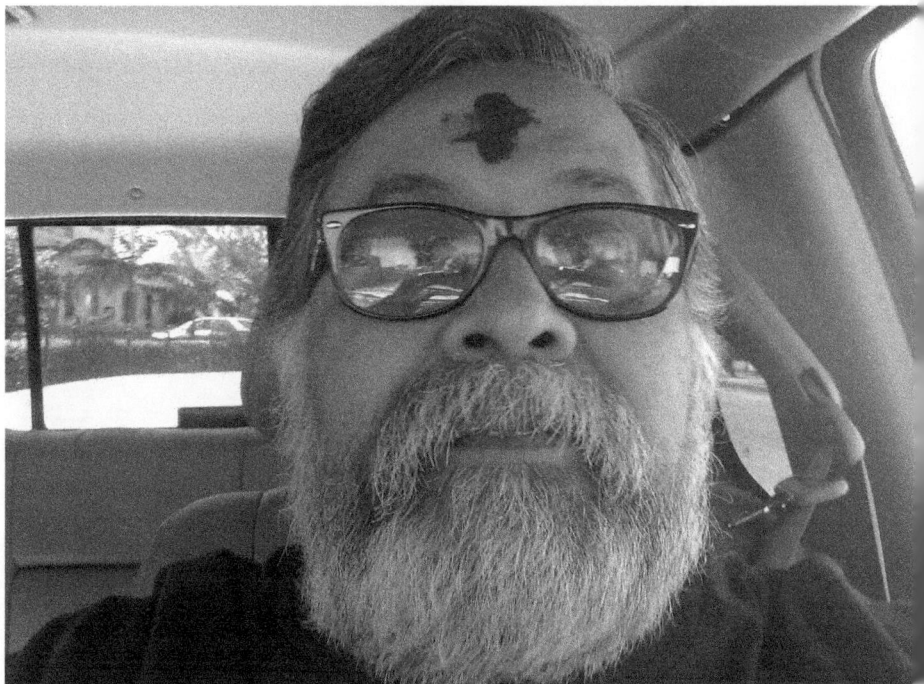

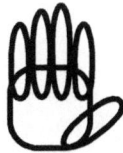

Part III: All Apologies

Let Me Apologize – February 13, 2013 1:19 A.M.

When I last posted, I left off right when I found out that I had a fistula in my urethra…but first, let me apologize.

I apologize for any confusion you might have up to this point and probably after, regarding my last post. I received a few replies and thank you for your concern but all of that happened in August. I'm sorry for any confusion – I'm not that good at this blogging thing.

I'm trying to keep everyone updated with what I'm going through now and at the same time I am going back from the beginning and telling my story. Hopefully I can help someone in a similar situation – that's what all of this is about.

When all of this started, I tried to find someone who I could talk to about these things but I didn't have any luck. My exact situation was very uncommon. In fact, Dr. Gregory told me that she had only seen it once before in her 15 years of experience.

Anyway, regarding my urethra – I wouldn't see my urologist Dr. Norouzi for a few weeks but I was still seeing all my other doctors for follow ups. My oncologist, Dr. Mahmood is a very busy man so that visit went well but took two hours.

Sitting down for any extended time is not very comfortable; I'm wearing Depends with a feminine napkin to soak up all the stuff that's still draining from my surgery, and I have the Foley catheter and my wound from the front is still fresh and draining as well.

I'm a mess.

But I need to see these doctors, especially Dr. Mahmood. He has a plan. He is totally aware of how my surgery went and tells me what the next step will be.

I'm going to be doing six sessions of chemo every other week, (very similar to how I started) and every Wednesday I will be infused with a drug called Erbitux. He tells me that Erbitux will starve the cancer of oxygen and blood, literally killing the cancer.

Yes! Let's kill this bitch!

I want to start chemo as soon as possible and I get the feeling so does Dr. Mahmood. I tell him about the fistula and that Dr.Norouzi is thinking of putting another kind of catheter in me, a supra pubic tube. It will go directly into my bladder and the urine will not drain out through my urethra and that will allow the fistula to heal. But all this takes time and a lot of pestering on my part.

Meanwhile, I'm being cared for at home three times a week by the Home Health nurses. They change my colostomy bag and change the bandage on my front wound and check on the sutures on my rear. They check my blood pressure and ask me how my appetite is – they have a very thorough check list.

I get to know Keith and Bernice very well. Keith is becoming very concerned about my front wound; all the staples have been taken off and it's healing very well except for the last one closest to my pelvic area. It's consistently 8cm deep and it's not healing like the others.

My next follow up is with my radiologist, Dr. Robert Ash. I haven't seen him since mid-May when my radiation treatment ended and it's now early September. Dr. Ash is pretty cool, but brutally honest. I have learned to appreciate his honesty, which is almost rude, but I'd rather have it that way. Just tell me like it is, doc.

Like Dr. Mahmood he is also very up to date with the results of my surgery. I also tell him about the fistula. But this is just a follow up and there won't be any more radiation treatment.

When this appointment was made it was assumed that I would be back to work by now or close to going back, but things aren't working out that way…at all.

He gives me the once over, and then tells me that considering what I started with (meaning my tumor – it was 13-cm long and now it was barely 3-cm), he said Dr. Gregory did a great job. Also my lymph nodes were clean and my markers were good.

"You've done very well. A lot better than most."

Coming from him that statement had me walking two-feet off the ground. I felt so good when I left his office. After all that I had been through so far, to hear those words, I really needed that.

This period was probably my lowest point. I missed my high school reunion and I had really wanted to go.

I also missed a book signing at Cypress Park Library which included a great group of friends that I had met through Twitter and Facebook, but there would be other opportunities to visit.

I had to focus on getting all healed up, so I could start chemo, so I could kill this cancer, once and for all.

Chemo Session #5 – February 13, 2013 4:29 P.M.

Today I saw my oncologist, Dr. Mahmood. He's very happy with how my treatment is going. I have minimal side effects from all that I'm going through. I did get the flu a couple weeks ago but I'm over it now, thanks to the nurses in his office.

The flu is one of the worst things that can happen to someone going through chemo. My temperature was 101 but they took care of me. As soon as I said, "I have the flu..." they went into action. And other than being anemic I'm in pretty good shape.

So now the $64,000 question: How much more chemo will I need to go through?

And the winner is...12 sessions, total!

Dr. Mahmood said there's no real set amount of chemo sessions that I could have. Six might do the trick. Eight might do it. But he considers me young at 53-years old, and I do have the potential to live a long life. So why not do the 12 sessions and say we did everything we can rather than oops, we only did six and the cancer is back.

This is our best chance to kill the cancer right now and since I'm doing so well as far as being able to withstand all that they infuse me with, then let's go for broke.

No regrets.

He said he doesn't want to have to treat me later on down the road. He said if I was 70-years-old he would leave it at six sessions. All in all, I'm good with 12. I mean what was I supposed to say?

No! Six is my limit. Ha!

Yippee-kay-yay mother fucker!

Early September: Still Healing From Surgery – February 17, 2013 10:36 P.M.

Slowly but surely things are coming together. I have a fistula but now something else has to be dealt with: my wound in the front. Keith is going to recommend to Dr. Gregory that we use a wound vac to get that little hole to heal.

A Wound V.A.C. (Vacuum-Assisted Closure), for those of you not in the know, is a small box that sucks out all the crap that's inside of me and promote the wound to heal. It's slightly heavy and they tape a tube to the actual wound, and then use foam to get a good air seal. Sounds good anyway.

I told Dr. Norouzi, my urologist, that at night when I lay down to sleep I can feel the urge to pee, and I have a Foley catheter on, so I shouldn't be feeling these urges. My bladder is being over active and when it contracts and tries to work it squeezes urine into my urethra and out my ass.

So in the morning when I check myself, I'm still wearing Depends and at night I put paper towels inside to catch all that's coming out. So he gives me these VESIcare (solifenacin succinate) pills to calm down my bladder and they really work well.

My bladder stops putting urine out so things start drying up in my rectum area. Things are really starting to heal…except for the small wound and the fistula.

So I get the wound vac at the house and three times a week the nurses re do all the tape and everything. And I tell Dr. Norouzi that Dr. Mahmood wants to start chemo asap. So we need to get that supra pubic tube in me too, asap. Chop, chop.

I don't wait for phone calls. I try to keep all these doctors as informed as I can. Hopefully the wound vac and supra pubic tube can do their healing so I can start chemo. I tried to start chemo with all these contraptions but Dr. Mahmood said no way. He wants me 100-percent healed before we start the chemo.

Damn.

The procedure to install the supra pubic tube will be my third procedure where I'm put under. Before all this happened, I had never been put under in my life. But it's a simple procedure and I'm looking forward to losing the Foley catheter.

Yippee.

This is an outpatient procedure so it happens at another facility very close to St. Joseph Hospital. I'm practically a regular here. I see Dr. Gregory down the hall but I don't want to raise my voice and say: HI, DR. GREGORY!

Dr. Norouzi comes by for last minute instructions and the next thing I know I'm waking up in recovery. This time Dr. Gregory is there to say hi. She's so awesome. She leaves and in comes Dr. Norouzi – he's one happy camper.

"Look! Look-look-look! This is the smallest fistula I have ever seen!"

Dr. Norouzi is holding a sheet of glossy pictures of my fistula.

Hey now.

He is so proud of these pics but all I can think of is: you put a camera up my penis.

And he said a bunch more stuff and I kept thinking: you put a camera up my penis.

Huh.

Ok.

I have my supra pubic tube and according to Dr. Vorouzi my fistula should be healed in hopefully a few weeks.

It's so small. I have pictures.

So I have a wound vac that's sucking the crap out of me and a supra pubic tube that doesn't hurt as much as a Foley. There's still some pain but not as bad. Now we need time for all this to work.

And the healing continues…

Chemo has Been Kicking my Ass Lately – February 19, 2013 10:06 P.M.

It kicked my ass for sure last Friday. Took me by surprise! It just sneaks up on me and then, Bam! Pow! I'm down in the fetal position. Yeah, Friday was bad and now every day I can feel it trying to sneak up on me.

After five chemo treatments I've probably reached some point of saturation. It's to be expected. Up until now I've been like, "Hey, this game is easy…" Well, those days are over, Jack.

I like to describe chemo as getting on a rollercoaster and not being able to get off. Well, this is the part where you want to stop the rollercoaster and get off but nope, it's not going to happen.

I have seven more sessions to go so I better get somewhat used to this. Last Friday I smoked some weed and that helped but I also had a brownie laced with marijuana that I had been saving for an emergency.

I had purchased it about a month ago and threw it in the freezer. I was told just to eat a quarter or third of it, so I ate about a third and that was plenty. That brownie really packed a punch. And I'm glad because it completely eliminated the yucky, crappy feeling that chemo gives.

I do have two pharmaceuticals that I've been prescribed, and I take them every morning. They're for nausea. They work but I'm sure there's some sort of side effect so I use them in conjunction with the medical marijuana.

I just recently read in the OC Weekly about a marijuana cooperative that has tamales with marijuana – pineapple tamales with some Mary Jane?

Yes! I will try them. I need to renew my card. It expired last week.

Tomorrow is an Erbitux day.

Whoop.

Damn. Healing Takes Time – February 22, 2013 4:34 P.M.

That's why patience is a virtue. Otherwise…so where were we? July 26th was the surgery. I had a Foley catheter for eight weeks then a supra pubic tube for almost six weeks and then I carried around a Wound V.A.C. for five weeks. So it must be November.

The tubes for the Wound V.A.C. and the suprapubic catheter tube are very close to each other, not more than three inches apart.

So I can't start chemo until I lose the Wound V.A.C. and the fistula is healed. Dr. Mahmood insists that I'm 100-percent healed so there will be no possible infections from any open wounds.

The fistula, according to Dr. Norouzi, was almost healed when the supra pubic tube was inserted. So hopefully that will be the first to pass the heal test.

Four weeks after the procedure, Dr. Norouzi sets up a test to see if the fistula is healed. It's the same test I had to take in order to find the fistula. I have to have a Foley catheter put on so they can fill my bladder with a liquid contrast then take some x-rays.

Yeah, sounds easy.

My bladder hasn't been stretched out in three months (red flag). The test is done at The Pavilion at St. Joseph. There's a doctor, a tech and a nurse. The doctor is asking me my medical history so he knows what he's looking for. He'll be taking the x-rays and I'm explaining to him about my fistula. The tech is getting things ready for the nurse whose job is to put the Foley catheter on me.

She tells me to take a deep breath, and before I can breathe deep, it's wham bam thank you ma'am and there's your Foley catheter.

OUCH.

Mean old nurse.

Meanwhile, the doctor is still asking me questions and I'm doing the best to answer while they start to fill my bladder with the contrast liquid. It doesn't take long when I say: OK my bladder is full...

And the doc says: But we need to fill enough liquid in order for this test to work.

Oy.

More liquid.

More anxiety.

I'm having flashbacks to when the Foley was plugged and the nurse had to come to the house but it took her 45 minutes to get there and I'm starting to freak out.

The doctor asks me about my rectum and I say I don't have one.

"They didn't leave you an anus?"

"No. But feel free to look…and can we hurry with this test, I have to pee!"

So the doctor has to check my ass to see that, hey, there's no butthole.

Wow.

Ok.

Let's take some x-rays!

The doctor is done so the tech can now take off my Foley…but where's the extractor?

Oh, it's locked up in that cabinet.

So where's the key?

Oh, it must be in the office…

HURRY!

Damn.

As soon as he released the Foley I voided right on the table but they had put towels around me. Still, I made quite the mess.

Now all I can think about is that I better pass this test because I cannot or will not go through this again. It's too much. I'm done.

And…yes!

The fistula is healed! Yay!

We leave the supra pubic tube in my bladder but we plug the end of it and this will allow my urine to come out the normal way.

Finally.

And it does. It works. But meanwhile we won't remove the supra pubic tube for a few weeks to make sure there's no leakage.

No problem.

That leaves the Wound V.A.C. and my small, little (now) 7-cm deep wound. Finally the main home health nurse is convinced the wound vac isn't going to work so Keith asks Dr. Gregory what's next. She says silver nitrate.

I'm like, "And then what ? Voodoo? Santeria?"

Silver Nitrate didn't work, so now Dr. Gregory has to go back in and find out why this wound isn't healing. Like Keith says, two steps back to go forward.

I've been saying, you should have done this five weeks ago!

Now for some more surgery – my fourth procedure this year.

Dr. Gregory finds a rogue suture that wouldn't dissolve. That's what was holding up the healing process. As soon as this is healed (and it took about three weeks) I will close the books with Dr. Gregory and let Dr. Mahmood take over with the chemo and Erbitux.

December 2011 is when I was diagnosed with cancer and now it's December 2012 and I will be starting 12 sessions of chemo and 24 sessions of Erbitux.

I originally thought this would take six months tops and I would be back to work. Not even close.

Chemo Session #6 – February 27, 2013 9:42 P.M.

Well, this was supposed to be my last treatment but as I stated in my last post I will now be doing 12 sessions of chemo. But doing 12 doesn't mean I need to do 12, it's mostly preventive maintenance.

It's also not official but from what Dr. Mahmood told me, if I was tested now I would probably be negative for cancer.

And that statement has slowly sunk in over the last two weeks.

I'm cancer free!

Unofficially.

I'm No Crash Test Dummy! – February 27, 2013 7:02 P.M.

Last week, while I was getting my Erbitux on I was approached by St Joseph Hospital to be part of a study for a new vaccine. My oncologist felt that I would be an ideal candidate.

I listened to the spiel and said I would think about it.

So, today as I was getting chemotized, they came back at me to try and close the deal. I listened and politely declined but they kept up the sales pitch and I said: NO.

The vaccine was for shingles and I had a 50/50 chance of getting them.

Shingles!

Fuck that!

Tengo cancer. No quiero shingles.

And that was the Basic Story – March 25, 2013 – 12:13 A.M.

I have told you from my diagnosis until now the basic overall story and experience of the last year, but I did leave out some stories. Not on purpose, mind you, but just so I can give them the time that these stories deserve. And as I learn more I would like to share my knowledge with others that are going through colostomies and radiation and chemo and dealing with everything else like insurance, friends and family.

Considering the cards I was dealt; stage 4 colorectal cancer, I consider myself lucky. Things could definitely be worse. I never lost my hair (even though I was prepared to) and could give a crap if I did.

I've lost some weight but my appetite has been good throughout. I did have some diarrhea but I've yet to throw up. Last week my calcium was low – that was a first, so I had to go get "calciumed" up: a two-hour drip. No biggie.

On the flipside, some people just have the worst time with treatment. Some people even refuse to go through treatment because of what they've heard that chemo will do to you. They choose to go with a more natural route. I don't know about that – everyone who I have heard that did this has died. But I'm sure there are some that survive and that's great.

I believe in science and am glad I've taken my chances. It's borderline torture but I am alive and after I'm done with my 12 chemo's I hope to live a long time.

If anyone has any questions, I will do my best to answer them. There's so much information out there. The internet has been good to me. I've met some awesome gente. On Twitter, I follow some great writers with cancer who tell it like it is.

I recommend to anyone with or without cancer to read what they're writing about daily: @xeni, @suleikajaouad and @adamslisa.

If you have cancer or know someone with cancer you're not alone…as long as I'm here.

A Story from my Stay in the Hospital – March 10, 2013 9:38 P.M.

Even though I was in the hospital only eight days, a lot went on. Learning about my colostomy was one of the most important lessons I was to learn. There were two ostomy nurses that came to my room to teach me how to change my bag. My sister Denise was there to help me and also to learn.

They came on a Monday and showed us the basics of how to take off the old bag and then put on a new one. When they came back on Wednesday I apologized to the nurses because I didn't remember a thing they'd said on Monday. But they were super nice about it and we pretty much did the same thing that we did on Monday.

I can't remember their names but the ostomy nurses were really nice. They offered to call in a volunteer, either a man or a woman, to help.

The man had a colostomy and was very physically active. They told me he worked out, he golfed and skied etc. and that he would come in to talk to me and answer any questions.

The woman had an ileostomy and she was the President of the Ostomy Association of Orange County. An ileostomy is when the small intestine is diverted where as a colostomy is where the large intestine is diverted. They both come out of a small opening in your abdomen, usually the lower left side. I went ahead and picked the woman. Her name is Teri.

Teri called me to arrange a time to visit. Of course anytime was fine by me, all things considered. Teri came by in the afternoon around the lunch hour so my family was there and so were a couple friends, Mike Schmidt and Diana Espinoza.

She brought some pamphlets and other sources of information. She told us all about her experience with her ileostomy and she was really a wealth of information. You can read books and search the internet but when a person with real world/life experience comes by to help with your transition? Wow, I was so grateful.

And Teri really was so helpful. After she told us her story she opened it up to questions and while I had plenty I'm so glad my family and friends were there because they also had some very good questions. It was definitely one of the high points of my hospital stay.

The Ostomy Association meets every month but because of the complications of my recovery and now I'm doing chemo, I haven't yet joined or attended a meeting. But I'm looking forward to one day joining my fellow ostomites where I'm sure I will continue my ongoing education.

Aja – March 11, 2013 9:10 P.M.

While rummaging through my storage unit I found a Steely Dan CD in pristine condition: Aja. I've been listening to it all day. Brilliant album!

I was in my storage to check out my fridge. Now that I'm smoking meat I need a fridge just to prepare said meat. It takes bacon a week to cure before you smoke it.

I was on Craigslist the other night and punched in: Kegarator. A fridge converted to a Kegarator popped up for $100, ready to go but I didn't pull the trigger. I know, I know…

I saw my radiologist today, Dr. Ash. It was just a follow-up.

Thumbs up.

See you in six months.

Yeah!

Earlier I felt like drinking a beer, then chemo set in. Yuck. I'm nauseated. So I pulled out the pot and started listening to Steely Dan.

History does repeat itself…

Chemo Session #7 – March 15, 2013 2:17 P.M.

This past Wednesday was my seventh chemo and 14th Erbitux sessions. So now it's all downhill from here. I have to do 12 and I projected that May 22nd should be THE DAY!

Then, hopefully, I can get back to work. I'm not even on the dole, I'm on my own. My disability ended in December and I've had to pay for my benefits thru Cobra. It's all good.

We can't plan our cancer treatments. I thought six months tops and I'd be back to work. If I can get back by June 1 then it will be a year and a half that I've been out of work.

But I'd do it again if it meant saving my life.

No question.

Everything happens for a reason. When I was going through a divorce, I moved back in with my mom and brother in order to get my financial house in order. I always insisted that "I'm just visiting" but that was, oh about nine years ago. So I'm in a very good place, to say the least.

Wednesday's treatment went as usual except around noon a new Pope was elected. As a Catholic in okay standing, I am interested in who will be leading this flock of diverse Catolicos. White smoke! Woo hoo! And the winner is…Argentina/Italy. Good luck, new Pope.

I did need to get a Procrit[6] shot because I'm anemic. Other than that I also got a visit from the physician's assistant, Esther Lamb. She was asking how I feel and the usual questions; any pain? No diarrhea? No headaches? No shortness of breath?

No.

She said after my 12th session I will be getting a PET scan. After that, I hope to get my clean bill of health.

I felt good after this treatment, but I still went home, ate some cereal, rested and then ate half a pot brownie.

Whew.

Good stuff…

---

6   Procrit is a prescription medicine used to treat certain types of anemia

Comfortable Places, Comfortable People – March 24, 2013
3:14 P.M.

After I got my diagnosis, my initial thoughts were to tell my family and friends but in what order? And what do I tell my mom? I started with my sister, Denise and then a couple of close friends. It's a hard conversation not only to have but how do you start it?

I think it's best to just cut to the chase.

When I got home I told my brother, Kevin, but I didn't tell my mom, not yet. I needed to know more about what I was going to go through. My mom needs to have facts so I waited a few days until after I met with Dr. Gregory. Then I would know more about what direction my journey would take.

As I was able to tell more family and friends I could tell that I would have some great support. Friends that I hadn't seen in years would contact me and talk about whatever they could do to help. Over time I would meet people with cancer on the internet, mostly through Twitter, and we would support each other. Still do.

I was building a small army of friends and family that would inspire me to get through the worst days of treatment. I felt safe with these friends. And that's a great feeling when you have cancer.

At this time, my safest, most comfortable place was going to be my room. The first thing I did was buy a 47-inch LG flat screen TV and set it up with Netflix. Going through the initial rounds of chemo and then six weeks of radiation, all I could do was watch TV.

My immune system was being ravaged so I needed to stay away from the general population. I was almost like the bubble boy; I wouldn't even go to see a movie, my favorite thing to do during the day. I would do my shopping either very early or very late, right before the store closed in order to avoid people. I couldn't afford to get sick.

Between the end of my radiation treatment and my surgery I had some time to recover and build my strength for surgery. I started to venture out a little, to some comfortable places.

If any of these places seem a little weird all I can say is that it's not so much about the place itself but the people who work at these establishments, for they are the reason I find certain places comfortable.

And I feel it's important to have these places in your life, whether you're sick or not.

For years my friends and I have been watching Monday Night Football, Laker games, Angels games etc. at the Alcatraz Brewery. I guess it's our hangout.

On my own, I decided not to drink alcohol during my chemo treatment. I figured I should give my body the best chance to fight the cancer and drinking would probably inhibit the way chemo could do its job. So when I told Mark, the manager, the bad news about my cancer and I was going to go through chemo, so he wasn't going to see me for a while, he was so nice and insisted that I still stop by if I was up to it and watch the games. He would message me and ask how I was doing and could he buy my dinner? Anything to get me out of the house and restore a little sense of normalcy.

So sure, I would take him up on his offer but mostly I knew that I could just go and hang out, relax, with a nice group of people. That was important. Steve, Jono, Charese, Rene, Alex, Jacie, Shane, the bartenders and servers, all great people, always making sure I was alright.

My favorite library isn't in Santa Ana, it's in Cypress Park. I feel so comfortable there that I think nothing of driving from the OC to the OG. And if I can't make it to see a certain program, they put it live on the internet.

Through Twitter I met the librarians, Art, Alicia, Patrick and the heckler. Art organizes programs that are sometimes geared for the kids and sometimes for adults, different speakers or authors – they have what they call 'Open Mic' night. Anyone can show up to read poetry or sing a song. I think it's very important for the community to have these programs. The lectures given by author Gustavo Arellano are always highly entertaining, to say the least. Artist Lalo Alcaraz has been there to show his art.

Next month I'm looking forward to a visit at the library by author/publisher Santino J. Rivera.

I don't know what your library is up to these days but hopefully they're doing a great job like what's going on in Cypress Park.

Trying to get through this journey hasn't been easy but being surrounded by comfortable people in comfortable places has really helped. We all have them.

Chemo Session #8: Yuck – March 29, 2013 9:35 P.M.

Yeah. Yuck times 20. Whew. Going into chemo I was feeling GREAT. I had just spent four days down in Playas de Tijuana with my brother Jeff and his buddies. I had never been to Playas but was impressed with how laid back it was. Considering it's a mere 10-minutes from the insanity of T.J. it's very low key.

They have a beachside boardwalk with plenty of places to eat and drink but it seems to me, most tourists just bypass Playas on their way to Rosarito or Ensenada, which is great, as far as I'm concerned.

Jeff moved into a nice house in a nice neighborhood, walking distance to your essential places like the Caliente Casino and Sportsbook, Cineopolis, Starbucks, KFC, Carl's Jr. and the XOOX convenience store.

And yes, plenty of taquerias. ¡Ajua!

I came back refreshed and relaxed but chemo had other plans for me. I seem to get more nauseated and was unable to eat after chemo. It was very overwhelming. I don't throw up…yet. It was just super yucky.

So I turned to my medical marijuana to take the edge off and then onto to Noble Ale Works for a few beers (despite swearing off alcohol previously), three to be exact. Another comfortable place.

I still never ate, which is OK, I guess. I purposely gained weight, once my appetite got back to normal, after I finally recovered from my surgery. I had lost weight after my first round of chemo and radiation and then lost more weight after my surgery. So going into these last 12 rounds of chemo I felt better being a little heavier and so did my doctors.

I didn't want to assume that because I did so well with the first round of chemo and radiation that I would do well with the second. And by that, I mean, it could have been worse, way worse! But I survived, like Dr. Ash would say, better than most, considering everything.

But those first rounds really did beat me down, way down and then my surgery kicked my ass. With all the complications that followed, I was unsure what was left of my resolve and what more my body could take.

So I ate.

And I got healthier.

The complications from my surgery and the delay that followed allowed me to get strong and healthy for the 12 rounds of chemo. Everything happens for a reason, right?

Well I believe in that.

Four rounds left and then I'm done.

Finished.

And I'm going to work hard to lose this weight, after all I've been through, losing weight should be a piece of cake!

Chemo Session #9: It's Not a Marathon but it Sure Feels Like One – April 9, 2013 4:47 P.M.

Tomorrow I will go through with my ninth chemo session and 18th Erbitux drip. I can almost see the light at the end of the tunnel. No, not that light! You know what I mean.

I consider myself very lucky. Hopefully sometime in June I will be back at work. That should be interesting.

Yesterday I started to clean the garage and I lasted 45-minutes. I was pooped. I showered and then took a two-hour nap. So I hope I can handle an eight hour work day. Real work! Soy Carnicero[7]. ¡Ajua!

I try to maintain a "normal" as possible life every day. I do chores, try to read etc. but it's getting harder to maintain a normal level of concentration.

Chemo brain. I got it. Bad.

I haven't been able to write anything in a while. I have the ideas and plenty of stories but I turn on my laptop and usually pass out. Of course, my problems are minimal compared to others.

Going back to work is going to be great but I already know I'm going to miss hanging out with my mom. It hasn't been easy for her, watching me go through all of this, but at the age of 87 she is an amazing person. I still learn from her. She has much knowledge and wisdom.

7   Butcher.

She watches me like a hawk. When I couldn't cook for myself she was there making hard boiled eggs for me or just getting me some cereal. At first she wanted me to get well as soon as possible. No one knew it would take this long to kick cancer's ass. So she was a little impatient with me. I never lost my hair to chemo and I lost some weight but not much so I always looked OK. She would look at me like, are you really sick? why don't you go to work?

But she got used to me "not doing anything."

I think after my surgery we all realized how bad my cancer actually was. Everyone really pitched in to help. I was a mess. But as I got stronger, I was able to help out with the cooking, the grocery shopping, you know, easy stuff.

We eat our dinner in the living room, watching the news, usually. Then at 7 p.m. she starts to watch her novelas. This is the highlight of the day. Those novelas are crazy! Boobs everywhere. Drama, drama, drama! And everyone is crying, always with the crying, and the boobs.

So we just sit back and watch these shows play out and laugh. I love to watch my mom laugh. I can see her as a little girl growing up in Stanton, having the time of her life even though she grew up during the Depression.

She was the youngest of 12 kids - the baby, that's what her friends called her. She was so small. Her name is Hortense, not Hortencia.

Never, NEVER call her Hortencia.

Erbitux Drip #19: Just Woke Up – April 17, 2013 7:22 P.M.

The last 24-hours have been brought to you by chemotherapy. Pow. Last night I felt pretty bad but I slept well. When I woke up though, I felt like someone had worked me over; you know, beat up, tired, sore. I usually wake up and I'm ready to go, and for the record, I don't drink coffee. This morning was bad.

I had an 8:45 am appointment for my Erbitux treatment. I didn't want to miss that so I did my best to wash up and get out of the house and on the road. I made it on time and told the nurse how I felt. She said that it's to be expected and she drew blood to make sure I wasn't too anemic. I tested fine. Yay.

I slept through the whole treatment. That's never happened before. I felt good after I got out of treatment. No nausea, still tired but I was hungry!

I called the compa[8] and we had lunch at Willowick; very good and convenient and right by the house. So I said thanks, went home and slept…I just woke up. And I feel great! Whew.

Last week, I had the full chemo treatment number nine and I had another visit with my oncologist. Nothing but good news. My blood work is good. Tumor markers, liver function, I'm still a little anemic but that's what blood transfusions are for, or the more common Procrit shot. And that's exactly what the nurse gave me.

I did mention to the doctor that when I attempt to exercise, which in my case is walking farther than my room to the fridge, that my feet tend to get swollen. I know it's from the chemo; I'm just worried how it will affect me when I go back to work.

The doc told me to wear high compression socks and to keep my feet elevated. It will take time for the long term effects of chemo to wear off – a long time – but eventually it will.

Other than my weekly chemo treatments I try to maintain as normal a life as possible. It was my brother Jeff's birthday recently and we had a good time celebrating. I smoked some ribs, chicken wings and smoked a couple of slabs of bacon. We went to an Angels game too (boy they suck!) It's going to be a long season.

But days like yesterday and today remind me that I still have about two months of treatment left and I will have some bad days of fatigue and nausea.

A small price to pay to be cancer free.

The Radiation Torture Marathon – May 2, 2013 12:50 A.M.

Today was my 21st treatment for Erbitux. It went very well. I had the new nurse and she was not only great but super-efficient. She had me out of there in less than two-hours. So, I was feeling pretty good when I left and that's how I always feel considering they just pumped me full of toxic chemicals. I did need another Procrit shot but I was this close to

---

8   Short for compañero, aka dude, friend, homie.

needing a blood transfusion.

This close.

Chemo is starting to really get to me. I'm sleeping a lot in the afternoons. After my treatment I saw my good friend Frank Martinez and he was taken aback by the condition of my skin. I use lotions and Aveeno soap but after five months and now 21 treatments it's dried out, puffy and discolored. And that's the skin you can see!

I have to go back to the oncologist office tomorrow because in my toxic daze, I forgot to ask for refills on my anti-nausea meds. Duh. And I need to get a doctor's note to go back to work. The girl that writes the notes wasn't there. D'oh!

Exactly a year ago at this time I was finishing my radiation treatment: six weeks of torture to save my life. And it did. No regrets. But if there was any time during my year and a half of treatment, it was that moment when I was mentally DONE.

I vividly remember telling the nurse or someone else that I didn't think I could finish. Being mentally strong had gotten me this far through all of the physical torture of radiation and chemotherapy. The radiation finish line was about a week away and I was on empty. And now you're probably waiting for me to say I had a miraculous apparition or some big time pep talk from some big time athlete that heard about this cancer kid…

No, this isn't one of those movies or stories.

I just kept showing up. I kept saying my Hail Marys and I kept asking all of you, my family, my friends, for support.

And I finished.

The Radiation Torture Marathon was done.

There is a picture of me at this time last year – I'm riding in a golf cart with Liliana, my goddaughter. She was practicing for the annual Cinco de Mayo golf Tournament at Willowick, of course. In the picture I have a huge beard and I'm smiling. Liliana brings great joy to me. She's on the golf team at Foothill High School. She kicks ass.

I'm glad her Dad will defer to me if Lili need's a certain golf club that her teacher suggests. It keeps me involved in her life and I would like to think that we both need that.

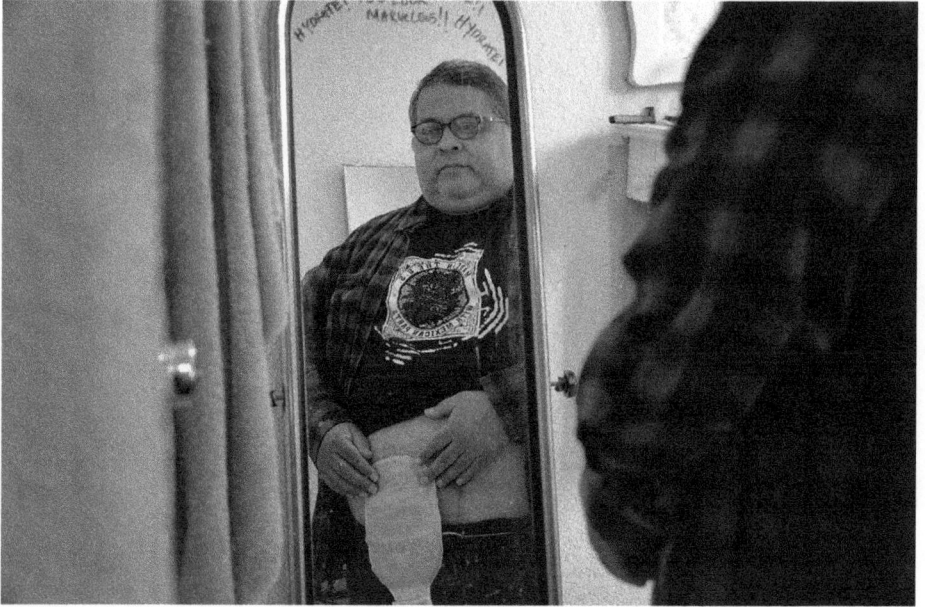

∞

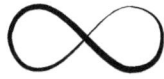

Part IV: The End & Beginning

Chemo Session #10: Q&A with Robert Flores – April 25, 2013 2:59 P.M.

As I approach the last two chemo sessions, I allowed myself to be interviewed by myself…

Q: So when is your last chemo session? And are you excited about going back to work?

A: Yes! My last chemo will be on May 22nd and on May 24th they will remove my chemo pump for the last time. Then I will start work – baby steps at first, but yes I am very excited to go back to my job.

Q: Will you have any testing done to determine if you are cancer free?

A: Yes. I expect to have either a CT Scan or a PET Scan, then when I get the results it will be official…cancer free! Yippee-kay-yay, mother fucker!

Q: How are you feeling right now? Can you put in an eight-hour day at work?

A: I told my district manager that I have zero stamina. I had to be truthful. This is my week: On Wednesdays I have treatment and I don't usually sleep for two days but then on the weekend it all catches up to me. By Tuesday I feel pretty normal, only to start the cycle again on

Wednesday. But by going back to work, I should establish the schedule that I was on for over 30-years. Work hard. Play hard.

Q: Sounds great. You're almost done after one year and four months. Anything else new going on for "Robert The Bold"?

A: Why yes, funny you should ask. My good friend from Florida, Santino J. Rivera, author/publisher, has offered to put my experience with cancer in book form. Part of the proceeds will be donated to a children's cancer foundation.

Thank you Santino for all your support, from day one you stepped up and sent me two of your poetry books. I took them with me to my first chemo sessions, back in January of 2012. I couldn't put them down and had to slow down when I read them. You opened my eyes and mind to what poetry could be. With your talent, I hope you can put my thoughts and words into a book worthy of all the cancer patients who are looking for answers.

It's one thing to get advice from your doctors, and I have nothing but respect for my doctors, but to be able to get answers or advice from a fellow cancer survivor makes a big difference and that's all.

What I want to do now, is help someone, anyone that is struggling with their cancer diagnosis. I never found a mentor when I got my bad news and that would have really helped me as I went from chemo to radiation to my surgery then recovery and 12 more chemo sessions. I learned a lot the hard way. But I'm alive and well. I beat the odds.

Stage 4 cancer is almost a death sentence. It has a 6-percent survival rate. Over 50,000 people will die this year from colon cancer. I hate these stats but they're real, as real as my story.

Let's do this.

Chemo Session #11: The end of one Journey and the Beginning of Another – May 11, 2013 11:59 P.M.

In two weeks, I'll go through my last chemo session, knock on wood. I'm having moments of overwhelming emotion. The last year and a half has had many memories; some good, some great and some that I'd rather not remember.

But that's why I started this blog...on the off chance that anything I've written might help someone going through cancer or that you might know someone with cancer and can pass along my experience.

For instance, last week, I had my treatment for Erbitux on Wednesday and got about four hours of sleep over three days. Now that really sucked. This week I had the full Erbitux plus chemo treatment and slept pretty well on Wednesday and almost all day on Thursday. What the Hell?

I figure after I stop treatment, it might take about a month to get my sleep pattern back to normal. I never used to have bouts of insomnia. Getting back to work will also help with a normal night's sleep.

Aha! Getting back to work…

I really have no idea when I'll be able to get back but I'm hoping that it's soon. I'll have a discussion with my oncologist not only about work but about what other tests and follow up visits that he'll want me to have.

So as I end this part of my life with cancer a whole other journey will begin: to heal my body from what saved my life.

One More Week, Two More Sessions – May 14, 2013 9:18 P.M.

Yesterday, I ended up at my primary doctor's office with the flu. I originally called my oncologist but they were booked, being Monday, so they suggested I call my primary, Dr. Lin. Good suggestion.

He had an opening at 10:30 a.m. Perfect. I think the world of Dr. Lin. He made the initial diagnosis of my cancer. I swear, I thought he was going to cry when he told me. I felt like giving him a hug. That was a year and five months ago.

"Seems like yesterday," he told me.

Now he smiles when he sees me.

He knows.

And that day, in December 2011, he knew what I was in store for. He knew what stage I was and that it would be a long road to kill this cancer. Everyone reacts differently when they're told they have cancer. Some cry, some go into denial, but we're all allowed to react as we do.

Since I thought Dr. Lin was going to cry, I gave myself about 10 seconds to think about it then I asked him, "So what do we do now?"

This was a Monday, December 12th to be exact, and Dr. Lin had already made arrangements for me to have a CT Scan on Tuesday and for me to meet with Dr. Anita Gregory, my surgeon, on Wednesday.

He was on it.

Sense of urgency.

My whole world changed in an instant. Things were happening very fast, and justly so. Dr. Lin picked Dr. Gregory and in turn she brought Dr. Ash and Dr. Mahmood on board, my Dream Team.

I will always appreciate Dr. Lin's sincerity, his sense of urgency and for choosing Dr. Gregory.

I wore myself out this last week; hockey game, compadre's birthday drinkfest, Mother's Day, smokeapalooza. I tend to lead my life not thinking I'm fighting a battle against cancer. I also tend to forget that I've endured 11 sessions of chemotherapy and 22 sessions of Erbitux in the last six months. It's just my way of letting cancer know that I'm in charge here. I'm the Boss.

Sure I have my bad days. I have side effects of all the chemo. And it sucks. But after next week, no more chemo – I'm done. I win.

But first I have to get over this flu. My immune system is shot.

Dr. Lin prescribed me Tamiflu. This stuff works great. I already feel better. Thanks Dr. Lin.

Thank you for everything.

Yesterday's Erbitux Session Went Well, Thanks to Dr. Lin – May 16, 2013 8:11 A.M.

I have two more sessions of chemo left, yesterday's session and then next Wednesday's. In order to see the oncologist, you have to make an appointment, so I made one for next week with Dr. Mahmood, but he was already booked so I get to see his P.A., Esther. She's pretty nice. I've seen her many times once I realized it was a lot easier to book her than Dr. Mahmood.

You make an appointment with him and he'll show up, eventually. With Esther, she's always on time and if she doesn't have the answers, she will track down Dr. Mahmood and ask him, so it's almost like seeing him but without the wait.

So yesterday, everything was dripping down just fine when Esther walks into my room. The rooms are very nice, individual with a nice little flat screen with cable, a comfortable recliner and some of the rooms even have views.

I was surprised to see her since, she was scheduled for next week and I wasn't prepared with all the questions I was going to ask her. She started to ask me about my skin. The Erbitux has really irritated it to the point where it's driving me nuts and my eyes are all fucked up. My eyelashes are almost all gone from me taking all the scabs out of them. Erbitux makes you break out with what looks like acne and pimples but when you pop one of these pimples blood comes out, not that white junk. Yuck.

I showed her my left leg which is covered with scabs as is my stomach and we had basically the same conversation I had with Dr. Lin on Monday. Hmmm...

On Monday my blood pressure was elevated and we talked about it. I told Dr. Lin that I know I had gained some weight but what was really bothering me constantly, was my skin. I was probably in pain but over time you get used to the pain and I do have a high tolerance to it, especially after all I've been through.

I always mention my issues to the nurses when I go in for treatment. But I'm not a big complainer. I tell them my skin is bothering me a lot and it's up to them to help me or just tell me the usual.

"That means the Erbitux is working, we like to see that."

Okay, I get it.

Get over it, Robert. Shut the fuck up.

In early February, I told them I had the flu and they went into action and took care of me ASAP. So it depends.

After the Q&A with Esther, she prescribed me antibiotics for my skin and a Bacitracin Ophthalmic ointment for my eyes. I was also low on calcium so I had to stay an additional three hours for that drip. I wasn't prepared for that one.

As I walked out with my new prescriptions I was thinking that Dr. Lin must have called or emailed my oncologist. Why else would Esther show up without an appointment and act so concerned?

I used that eye ointment last night and in 45-minutes, wow, what a relief to my ojos. About time! I think I'm going to start calling Dr. Lin "Dr. Shaft," because he is a badass mother fucker!

Hey, I'm talking about...

Another Brick in the Chemo Wall – May 20, 2013 9:56 P.M.

I started to write this last night but I hit the chemo wall. Finally. Yep, I felt fine until around 10 p.m. then it started. And it overwhelmed me.

I got so nauseated I thought for sure I was going to throw up. Eleven chemo sessions and 23 Erbitux treatments and I've not gotten sick. Sure, I get pretty nauseated, but never to the point that I would lose my lunch. That's a pretty good streak.

But streaks are made to be broken right?

I didn't vomit but I did get diarrhea.

Whew. I said it.

Diarrhea.

My first time with a colostomy bag too.

Interesting.

I survived. Three days before my last chemo session and I get sick. I'm ready for this to be over.

So I get up this morning, my birthday morning, and I'm feeling a little tired. I was planning to drive down to San Diego to meet my brother Jeff and go to Hodads (free Burger for the birthday boy). And I remember that I need to renew my drivers license. Damn! I better get cracking.

Get up, yo. DMV here I come. And I cancel the SD trip. I'm tired.

Chemo has taken its toll on me.

I end up at the DMV in Costa Mesa and after an hour and a half, I've renewed my DL. And all morning, I'm getting birthday wishes from everyone. THANK YOU! So much…they made my day and kept me going. All day I'm getting messages. How awesome! You guys and gals rock! Being able to celebrate my birthday the same week that I'm finishing chemo is so overwhelming. I'm truly blessed.

But I think I'll take it easy this week. My immune system is shot. I'm always tired now. Aaaand I got sick. But all this could have happened months ago, so I guess I did pretty good. Hell. Yes.

For my birthday dinner I went to Knotts Berry Farm and picked up some of their fried chicken with all the fixings. He shoots! He scores! I had boysenberry pie, the whole shebang. Yeah.

Thanks everyone for the birthday wishes and for all your support. I'm honored and humbled…tears of joy…it happens a lot lately, and that, my friend, is a good thing.

Chemo Session #12: Epic Fail – May 22, 2013 10:01 P.M.

I'm not a Negative Nelly, a Debbie Downer or a Wally-Wah-Wah by any means. Every morning I wake up and I'm one happy mother fucker. And today was no exception. Today was graduation day. My last chemo day. No mas.

My mom is a breast cancer survivor and on her last day of radiation, she gave her nurses boxes of See's Candies. I learn from the best so last week, I went to this bomb-ass bakery in Santa Ana to do some research: The Mill Bakery on Main Street. It's been there for years and they got the baked goods.

So I get up bright and early and go to the bakery to make my decision on what goodies to take to the nurses at the oncology office. It's a very large office with a lot of employees so I couldn't swing the See's Candy, that's why I was going with some sweet bakery goods.

I chose two beautiful coffee cakes, one for the front office and the other for the nurses in the infusion part of the office. After a year and a half of treatment, I've gotten to know everyone and everyone in the office knows me. I also picked up some pastries for the valet parking attendants. They work pretty hard and always have a smile on their face. I don't use the service but there are a lot of people that need it, like the elderly and those that are incapacitated.

So far, so good.

I punch in and wait to get called, and wait…and finally the nurse comes for me which is unusual because I'm there for chemo. Usually, I write my name down and they give me my order sheet and I go to the back where the infusion section is. If I'm supposed to see the Doctor, like today, they come in at their convenience. But I'm taken to a regular room and the nurse starts with the blood pressure and takes my temp.

"I'm supposed to be in treatment and I understand you're just doing your job but…"

So she goes back to the infusion center and the other nurses are like, where's Robert? So, she didn't know, no biggie, and I go back with my gifts of coffee cake to get the party started.

Woo hoo! My last chemo!

Let's start the drip! The sooner we start the sooner we finish. And boom! I knock out.

Cool. I've been up since 3 a.m. listening to Howard Stern anyway. I wake up and there's Diana Espinoza, my long-time friend from high school, and she's bearing gifts. It's some kind of treat from Starbucks's; she says it's salty with chocolate and caramel. Yes, I'm in a daze, but the visit is greatly appreciated.

Diana stays awhile and watches as the nurse changes the dressing of my PICC line. This happens every Wednesday. So Diana has to go and in walks Esther the PA. Dr. Mahmood was booked but Esther is very good and I have a lot of questions for her. I should have a PET Scan in about two weeks. Yay! And that should tell a lot, especially with my recovery.

Then she drops a bomb on me: One more Erbitux treatment next week.

NOOOOOOOOOOOOOOOO…

I don't ask why. If Dr. Mahmood feels I need one more then let's do it. It's not going to kill me, but cancer will. Everything else Esther and I talk about is a blur. It's all very important but I am slightly dejected. I'm bummed. I want to start detoxing ASAP. I want to get back to work

ASAP. I brought coffee cake!

I am very lucky. The side effects of chemo are many and I have been able to avoid the majority of them through these 12 chemo sessions. But for some reason the side effect of diarrhea has decided to make itself known in these last days of my chemo treatments. Not too long after Esther left, it started, and it was bad.

The infusion center is huge, so I go to a restroom way down the hall. And I'm in there for a while. The nurses finally come looking for me.

"I'm Okay."

"Alright…We were wondering because we haven't seen you in a while. Do you have Imodium at home?"

"Yes I do. Do you have any Imodium here?"

"No"

HUH?! I bite my tongue. The nurses are awesome and they do the best they can. It's not their fault that there isn't any Imodium in a place where they give you poison that causes diarrhea. But someone has made this decision not to have a box of Imodium in a place that they infuse poison into your veins and diarrhea is a major side effect.

Some patients have this side effect from the beginning of their treatment. Do they bring their own Imodium? There is a frickin' pharmacy in the building. This beautiful multi-million dollar building has Imodium for sale!

When I go back on Friday to have my chemo pump removed, I will bring a box of Imodium. I won't be a smart ass about it. I just hope it will be appreciated as much as the coffee cake was.

So Long Chemo Pump – May 26, 2013 12:46 A.M.

On Friday, May 24, my chemo pump was removed for the last time. Knock on wood. It was the end of a long relationship that started in January 2012. That's when my first six rounds of chemo started. I was diagnosed in mid-December of 2011.

My "Dream Team" of doctors made their recommendations for treatment and I'll never forget the day that I got the phone call from the nurse at the oncologist office to let me know exactly how my first rounds of treatment were to go down.

I was parking my truck at the Mainplace Mall when I got a call from Dr. Mahmood's office. I was just going to do some pre-Christmas shopping - just a quick run through to see what was out there. I wasn't planning on buying anything at this time because it was still too early.

Now, I was pretty gung ho after getting my diagnosis. I had already endured a colonoscopy, a CAT Scan and a PET Scan. Also, every doctor had given me the once over, if you know what I mean. They all wanted to see the tumor that rarely happens.

"Highly unusual," is all I heard.

And all I wanted to do was be the best patient I could be and I was mentally prepared for whatever lie ahead. Or so I thought...

I sat in my truck as the nurse began to tell me exactly what kind of chemotherapy I was going to endure. She went over the entire schedule of the infusion.

I was somewhat aware of various chemo treatments but still, to hear what the reality of my treatment was going to be was a little shocking. No, that's not completely true, I was completely numb as I listened to her tell me about how I would have to carry a chemo pump for two days. From Tuesday to Thursday, I would be connected to this pump. After five hours in the infusion center, they would connect me to a pump that would slowly infuse me with more chemo. Then on Thursday, I would go back and they would disconnect it. This would happen every two weeks.

BOOM!

Like a ton of bricks.

Reality really does bite.

I went into the mall and walked around in a daze, used the restroom at Macy's, wandered around some and then realized I left my phone in the restroom. Of course it wasn't there!

Well, if you're going to lose your phone, lose it in the mall. I went right over to the T-Mobile store and reported it lost and got a loaner and ordered a new phone. Whew. Two weeks later my chemo treatments began.

After I finished the six sessions of chemo I immediately went into radiation treatment. It was 28 sessions over six weeks and the whole time I would be connected to a chemo pump. 24 hours a day, 7 days a week, we never close, for six weeks, no break.

Now, carrying a chemo pump for two days isn't so bad. As far as bathing I could get by until they took it off and then take a shower. But then I had to figure out a way to shower with the chemo pump. Six weeks of this: wrapping my PICC line in Saran Wrap, then wrapping the chemo pump in a plastic bag and jamming it into the top of the shower curtain. It fit pretty snugly up there.

You do what you do, right?

So the chemo pump and I had quite a relationship. After my surgery I needed another 12 rounds of chemo, including the pump.

Aha! So we meet again, eh!

The next thing to go will be my PICC line. It's been in my left arm for a year and a half. That decision will be made after my PET Scan, then we'll know exactly where I stand.

My bloodwork is great.

My lymph nodes are clean.

One step at a time.

Fuck cancer.

Better Safe Than Sorry – May 28, 2013 9:11 A.M.

I was up early listening to Howard Stern interviewing Katie Couric. As usual it was a great and informative interview. I had forgotten that Katie's husband, Jay, had died of colorectal cancer at 42. 42! He was diagnosed and lasted only nine months.

At 42 there was really no reason to have a colonoscopy but you know what? It's never too early. One of my nurses at the oncologist had a colonoscopy earlier this year. She's in her early thirties. She saw some blood in her stool. Also, she told me that she's seeing more women in their late twenties and early thirties getting diagnosed with second and third stage colon cancer. So she wanted to make sure she was OK.

Her test came back negative for colon cancer and doctors

recommend having a colonoscopy at 50. I think it should be lowered to 45. The test is actually easy. It's the night before that's rough…when you cleanse your colon.

Talk to your doctor if you're in that age group. Get it done. Just do it. Better safe than sorry.

The Last Drip – May 31, 2013 7:07 P.M.

On January 17, 2012, I walked into Dr. Mahmood's infusion center to receive my first dose of chemotherapy. I was a little nervous but I had complete confidence in not only Dr. Mahmood but with all the nurses in the infusion center. The nurses would be the ones I would deal with for the majority of my visits. I only saw Dr. Mahmood a handful of times.

Before they actually hooked me up to the IV drip, I got a little orientation on the drugs they would be infusing and their side effects. Then the nurse hooked me up and left me to watch TV or read or whatever I could do to kill five hours or so.

Well I had a little prayer/speech/declaration prepared. I wanted this to be as positive an experience as possible. I had read about how some people just hated chemo and how some people even refused to go through chemo because of the side effects. I was 110% ready to go through with chemo and whatever happened to me, so be it.

If I lost all my hair, oh well, it would grow back.

If I lost weight, oh well, I could stand to lose some libras.

And everything else, I was told to just let them know and they had drugs to help me with whatever side effect that I had.

So as the first drips of chemo entered my veins I welcomed chemo into my body. I said:

Please do your job and kill this cancer. I know you will also wreak havoc on my immune system and I will be fatigued but I am prepared for the worst.

I felt that by having a positive attitude about chemo and enabling it to do its job, things would go as smooth as possible. And for the most part, it did.

I had some pretty rough days and a lot of pain. But at this point I had a lot of cancer to kill. And the process of killing this much cancer was very painful. Thank you Vicodin!

In addition to the cancer that surrounded my rectum, I had a tumor that came out through my skin which, initially, I thought was a cyst.

After about a month, that tumor got infected and boy, was that painful. One night I literally cried and prayed myself to sleep, the pain was so bad. I had never experienced so much pain and all I had at the time was over the counter Tylenol.

The next day, I went in to tell them and they prescribed me antibiotics and the Vicodin 500 ml, but that wasn't doing it either so they upped it to 750 ml. Ah, relief.

I had to pop one every four hours to keep the pain away. What was happening, was the tumor was dying, and breaking up and it got infected. So, this was a good thing. The tumor is what made my cancer a stage 4.

So, that's how it all started and now it has come to an end…for now. And I am asking Mr. Chemo to now leave my body and to make a graceful exit.

You did your job, my man. And I thank you. Go ahead, leave. Bye.

Adios…

Peeling Away at the Onion of Honesty – June 15, 2013 3:06 P.M.

In regards to a regular visit to the doctor for your annual checkup, the questions that will be asked by the doctor are usually answered with enough honesty but not enough truth.

The doctor will ask you: Have you been exercising? And of course you answer: Yes. Walking back and forth to the fridge is exercise, right? Have you been eating a healthy diet? And again you answer: yes, Dr. Lin, I eat all my veggies. Veggies being the tomato and lettuce on that Double Double we had last night.

And the doctor is fully aware of this chess game of Q & A. That's why he orders some blood work and sends you to the lab. Aha! Busted. Your cholesterol is high, your blood sugar puts you at the borderline of diabetes and your liver is showing the early signs if cirrhosis.

So now, when the doctor tells you that you have cancer, the degree of truth in your honesty changes…and drastically. Well, it should and for me it did. I went from the familiarity of my primary physician, Dr. Lin to meeting three doctors that would determine my treatment and my future. And one by one, you have these initial meetings.

With me, they all did a brief physical exam, they all wanted to see the "highly unusual" tumor. Then they sit you down and they have a whole slew of questions. I realized right away, the sense of urgency with my condition. As I would meet each doctor, I could also sense their interest was sincere, intelligent, along with the urgency to find the right treatment to kill this cancer.

We would meet one at a time and with the information they gathered from our meetings, they would get together to determine what would be the course of treatment. Things were happening very quickly. They were making the time to meet me. My oncologist, Dr. Mahmood stayed until after 6 p.m. to meet with me. So, on my end, I knew that I had to step up and be the best patient I could be, which meant answering their questions as honestly and truthfully as I could.

The onion was starting to be peeled.

Has your appetite changed? Have you lost any weight recently? How long have you had this cyst? How much blood is in your stool? How often do you go to the bathroom? Have any other relatives had cancer?

On and on it goes – each doctor with their questions. Some were the same but some were different. This was just the beginning.

Once I started with chemo the nurses took over. They also want to know things. How are you feeling? Anything bothering you? Let us know. You don't have to suffer. We can help with any side effect but you have to let us know.

And I did.

I didn't want to suffer. Hell no.

When I had pain I told them. Boom. Vicodin. Nausea. Bam. Zofran and Ativan. It was the same with going through radiation.

But all of this honesty can take its toll on a guy. As the layers and layers were peeled away I became more aware of my emotions. I wouldn't say I was unemotional as a person. I get choked up like most do when you go to a funeral or maybe when a movie scene is very sad. I'm not ashamed to say that I cry; not like a baby but more when I was overwhelmed by happiness.

After my surgery, when I came home, I was such a physical mess. At night, I would put on my headphones to listen to music and the first time I did this I cried…from happiness that I was alive. I cried that I had survived this damn surgery.

The surgery really made me realize how bad my cancer was. My iPod is full of all different types of music but it was the music of my youth – Stevie Wonder, Al Green – that got to me. It was as if I was hearing it for the first time. The words, the rhythms, it all seemed so brand new.

I felt lucky that I was given this chance to live. It was overwhelming and I did cry like a baby.

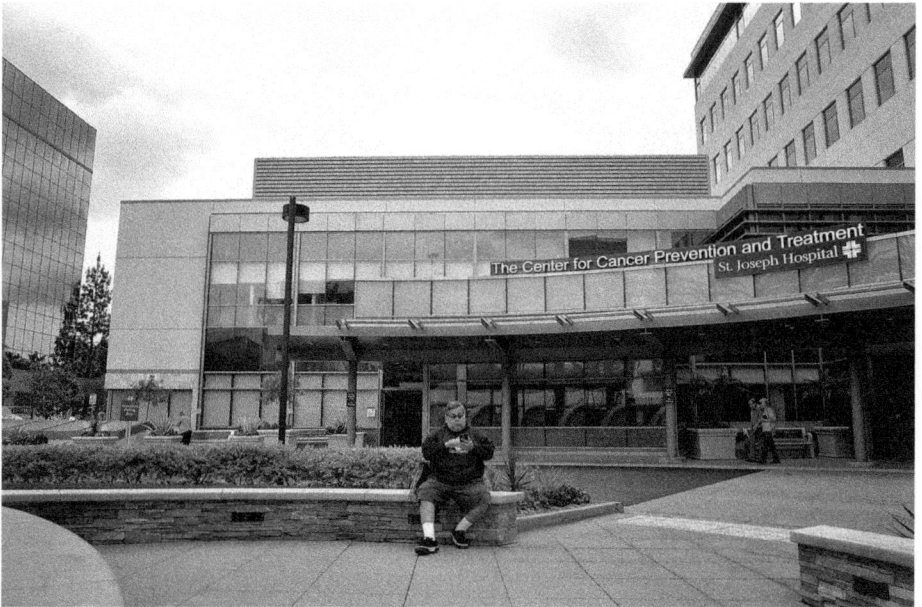

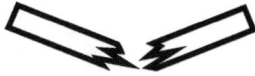

Part V: The Sweetest Revenge

Where Were You When You Found Out Robert Beat Cancer? – June 21, 2013 6:37 P.M.

After finishing my chemo and Erbitux treatments I was scheduled for a PET Scan for today, Thursday, June 20, 2013. A PET Scan uses a radioactive medicine known as a radiotracer to produce a 3-D image of the body. It's better than a normal X-Ray. My appointment was for 7:30 a.m . That made me the first patient of the day.

I've had this test before; it was last year about two months into my first round of chemo. They put that radiotracer into your veins; it takes about 45-minutes to an hour to settle into your body. It doesn't hurt at all. Then you go into the machine that is the same exact one they use for an MRI and CT Scans. It takes about a half-hour.

When the nurse was prepping me for the PET Scan I asked her when I could see the results. She said in usually 24-to-48 hours. I mentioned that I did have an appointment to see my oncologist, Dr. Mahmood later that afternoon and she made a note of that. I didn't get my hopes up because I could tell they were very busy.

The machine they use is fairly narrow and you are in there for about 25-minutes, but I'm not claustrophobic. They play very mellow music. It reminded me of middle earth; flutes and all. I was saying my Hail Marys to calm myself down. Smoking a blunt is out of the question.

As I was laying there, I had a moment of just knowing the test would go well. I started thinking of everyone that has supported me through this journey. Then, I started thinking of my abuelitas; my grandma Chencha and grandma Petra. Both have long passed but from the beginning, I prayed for to them to watch over me. I never really knew my abuelitos; one passed way before I was born and my Grandpa

Pete died when I was very young. You're supposed to remain completely still and here I was getting emotional and trying not to cry but the tears came anyway, happy ones.

I was going to be OK.

After the test, I came home and made a hearty breakfast for my mom and brother; sausage, papas and scrambled eggs with some bell peppers. I rested and waited for 3:15 p.m. and my appointment with Dr. Mahmood.

Dr. Mahmood is a very busy man and is notorious for making you wait, and wait and wait…but it's worth it. I check in and the nurse takes my BP and temp. She turns on the computer to log my vitals and sees that my PET Scan results are in.

Woo hoo!

I'm also scheduled to have my PICC line flushed, this is a weekly deal so another nurse from the infusion center comes in to flush my PICC line and change the dressing. She also draws some blood to check my white cells and red cells. After she's done, it's Dr. Mahmood's turn.

And I wait and wait and finally, his Assistant, Esther, walks in. She's going to take over because Dr. Mahmood is still busy with other patients.

No problem. Esther's cool.

She pulls up the PET Scan results and it's nothing but good news, strike that, GREAT news.

There are no signs of cancer.

Nothing.

Nada.

I'm done!

See you in three months.

Of course we talked about a lot more, like my PICC line, it will be removed next week. Yay.

Am I'm going back to work?

Yes, whenever you feel well enough.

Yay!

She gave me a copy of my PET Scan, which I plan on framing.

I call my compa to see if he was planning on watching Game 7 of the NBA Finals. I leave a message suggesting that we go to Tustin Brewery, but I don't mention that I'm cancer free. Then I think, wait a minute, Tustin Brewery? I should be going to Alcatraz Brewery, they have been so supportive, so awesome and beyond the usual.

So I call back the compa and start to leave another message but all I can get out is, "Let's go to Alcatraz…" and then it hits me like a 2 X 4.

Bam!

I AM CANCER FREE.

FINALLY.

I can't talk anymore because I'M crying, yes like a baby. All my focus for the last year and a half has been on kicking cancer's ass and I did it. But I wasn't alone in this battle. I had tons of support.

My mantra was: fuck cancer.

Cancer wanted to kill me and I said NO! And I'm not through fucking cancer.

Please follow my friend, Andrew on Twitter at @Amateurchemist. He writes a column about his fight with cancer at the OC Weekly. He is a badass cancer warrior. An inspiration.

Cancer is straight up evil. I hate cancer. No one should have to go through what I did. Kids get cancer every day. This has to end.

Fuck cancer!

A Brief History of the Colostomy – June 25, 2013 5:57 P.M.

I'll make this brief. Not so much because of cancer but mostly the problem (with crapping) back in the day was constipation. I'm talking severe constipation. Doctors were hesitant to operate on the intestines because a lack of antibiotics to combat the infection would surely infest an open incision in that area. To help "unblock" one's intestine, people used to eat mercury. The thinking was that the heaviness of the metal would push and clear the blockage. Even horseback riding was thought of as a solution.

Between 1716 and 1839, 27 primitive colostomies were attempted with only six survivors. And even at that, they only survived for a short time, usually only a few weeks. But perseverance always leads to success and now colostomies are almost routine operations.

Yay. That was brief.

I like to tell the doctors and nurses that my colostomy has been the least of my worries; especially after all I've been through. It hasn't been easy, but I've come to accept it. Of course what choice do I have? So I try to put the most positive spin on something that a lot of people have a hard time dealing with.

After I woke up from my surgery, I had to look to see if I really had the colostomy…

Yep.

It was there.

The nurse took care of it; emptying it, changing it. I didn't have to deal with it. I was a little scared even to look at it: my stoma (the part of the colon that is pulled through a hole in my abdomen).

Yeah.

It would take from four to five weeks before it would shrink down to its permanent size. After eight days in the hospital I was sent home and the Home Health nurses took over the care of my colostomy. I still didn't have to deal with it but I was watching and learning.

As I watched and learned to change the colostomy bag I got used to the stoma. And now I'm in awe of it. It's simply a miracle.

I thank those doctors in those pioneering days that knew that the colostomy would not only be the short-term answer but would allow people to live normal lives today and for many years to come.

It will be almost a year since my surgery: July 26, 2012. I'm very comfortable with my colostomy but I still have a lot to learn. My diet has a lot to do with how well I manage my colostomy.

Being on so many different drugs, whether it's pain pills or chemo toxins, has made it a little challenging. But all that's over, for now, and I should have normal bowel movements.

Also, I will be going back to work soon and that will also have a great effect on when I eat, what I eat and being more active will help as well. I'm looking forward to these new challenges.

Losing weight is on top of my new bucket list. I am nowhere near being 100-percent but I feel that by going back to work I will have a normal schedule which will lead to better sleep habits and hopefully everything else will follow.

Like life itself, living with a colostomy is what you make of it. In my case, because of the nature of my cancer and having the tumor compromise my sphincter muscle, I had to have it done. I was shocked and scared. I have to deal with it every day and at least six times a day I have to empty it. I thought I would never have to use toilet paper again but boy was I wrong.

You can't control when you will have a BM and I can let the bag get full and empty it twice a day but that's kind of gross. I empty it as soon as I need to.

My awesome ostomy nurse Keith told me, "This is your new rectum, Robert; you have to keep it clean."

And I do.

Going Back to Work – July 8, 2013 10:22 A.M.

I'm very excited to be going back to work this Tuesday. I'm nowhere near being 100-percent in shape for work but I felt that the best way to get in shape for work was to go back to work. I've been going to the gym and doing the treadmill but it's not the same as working.

It's going to take at least three months for the chemo toxins to completely dissipate from my body and last week I stopped taking the anti-nausea pills so that I could go through whatever withdrawal symptoms they might have. Mentally, I'm so ready for work but physically…time will tell.

All I can say is that the company I work for, Gelson's, has been nothing but supportive and great. Even my union made the comment that any other company would not have kept my job for this long (a year and a half).

They probably would have told me, "Sorry, we have to let you go, but when you get better, we will be more than happy to hire you back… of course, at the two tier wage and benefit package. Good luck!"

I've had but one profession in my life, I am a meat cutter and I love it. In high school, I played the sax and loved that too. When I was 16, I bought a Selmer Mark VI alto saxophone, arguably one of the best saxes in the world. I paid $300 for it and today on EBay they go for between $4,000 to $5,000. I still have it.

That would have been my first choice of employment. My junior year in high school, a friend, Henry Huizar, told me about a job at the meat market next to his work. Henry worked at a produce stand called The Potato Bin. I applied for the job and got it. I was working at Mel's Meats.

Mel's Meats was at one time a traditional meat market and a union shop. Times change and it now caters to the predominantly Mexican neighborhood, with thin cut meats for carne asada and tripe for menudo. It was a great after school job and I wanted to put in more hours.

I was playing sax in a band and making some money but I needed a steady job. I had to pay for my tuition at school. My parents divorced right before my freshman year so money was tight. I was first chair sax in Mater Dei High School's award winning band but I felt that it was time to quit and focus on school and work.

Unfortunately, the Dean at school wouldn't let me quit. I explained my situation at home but he didn't seem to care. In fact, he told me in no uncertain terms, "You won't make it through your senior year."

Excuse me?

Mater Dei is a great school. Myself and two other kids from my grade school scored in the top percentile when we took the entrance exam and entered Mater Dei with academic honors.

While both playing the sax and being in the band was a feather in my cap, I didn't need the band to get into Mater Dei. I couldn't quit the band, so I made the band quit me. I caused enough ruckus to get kicked out.

After I graduated, the owners of Mel's Meats told me that if I wanted to really learn how to cut meat, that I should move on, because they were limited as to what they could teach me. I found another job in Huntington Beach at J&R Meats. J&R was a gourmet meat market where I learned how to break down sides of beef, make sausage and how to really handle a knife. The owners were Jack (who owned a few markets called Sir Jax, which he sold to open this store) and Ron. Jack had learned to cut meat in Germany – very old school and a great guy. Ron was a younger man who had been a former apprentice of the year at Alpha Beta (another market).

Ron would eventually help me get into the apprenticeship program at Alpha Beta. He told me I needed to work at the big supermarkets where they cut meat in higher volume and that would help me become a better and more skilled cutter.

After I became a journeyman at Alpha Beta, I quit. Alpha Beta taught me to cut meat the "Alpha Beta way" and I knew there was still more to learn. I went to work at an independent market called Bell's California Farms. There I worked for Mike Robbins who taught me a lot. I then went back to work for the big supermarkets for the security of a union wage and the benefits.

I started working for Vons and even though I felt like I knew it all, it took a while to work my way up to meat manager. A Vons store manager, Dave Jones, was giving me a yearly appraisal and told me, "Robert, if you don't write down that you want to be a meat manager, I'm going to kick your ass."

I told him, "Dave, all I want to do is work 20 years for Vons and then work 10 years for Gelson's and retire a real meat cutter."

"You asshole," Dave said.

I did get promoted to meat manager, eventually got married and then in 2003 we had the epic supermarket strike. A lot was about to change. I was the shop steward and picket captain at my store and I did my best to maintain the best picket line for my coworkers. It was tough.

The strike would last for five months. Right away I decided to also get a part time job so I applied at Gelson's and got hired right away. Gelson's is a small chain of high end supermarkets with the same union as Vons. They sign what is known as a "sweetheart contract" to protect them from being the target of a strike.

Unexpected to the "big three" supermarkets, was the customer support of not crossing the picket lines. Gelson's business increased significantly. I was picketing in the morning and working at Gelson's in the afternoon and evenings. After the strike was over, the store manager at Gelson's told me that if I wanted to stay, I was more than welcome. But after 22 years with Vons, I felt an obligation to go back to Vons.

He left the door open, in case I wanted to change my mind. After two months, I did change my mind and called Hector, the meat manager, in Dana Point, and asked if I could come back. It took a month, but Gelson's took me back, under the old contract. I didn't lose anything in wage and benefits, other than my seniority with Vons and, of course, I wouldn't be a meat manager, but that was okay.

Giving my notice to Vons was like trying to quit the band at Mater Dei. Upper Management took me into the office and told me how I was making a big mistake, blah-blah-blah.

I told them that I wasn't quitting Vons, I was quitting Safeway. Vons didn't exist to me for quite some time after Safeway had acquired Vons and turned it into another corporate appendage.

I've been working for Gelson's for 10 years now, but I have no intention of retiring. About eight years ago, the opportunity to run the seafood department in Dana Point came up and I took it. My seafood department is one of the best in Gelson's. I love it.

Last week was the first week in a year and a half that I didn't have a doctor's appointment. Things are slowly getting back to normal.

One day at a time…

Going Back to Work…Continued – July 9, 2013 9:07 A.M.

I feel like it's the first day of school. I'm both nervous and excited. Last week, I talked to my meat supervisor and he told me to take breaks as I needed. He scheduled me for five days – 40 hours. I'm a full-time employee but he told me that if it was too much, to just tell him and he'll give me four days instead.

Gelson's has been awesome. Last night, it dawned on me, that I didn't have my safety glove. It's a steel mesh glove that we use (required by *OSHA), to protect us from slicing our fingers off. You have to have it or you can't work.

They scheduled me at the Newport Beach store to keep me closer to home, which is great. My home store is Dana Point, it's 25-miles one way. Right now driving that far is a bit much for me. Last time I went down there to visit, I was so tired by the time I got there. But that's where my mesh glove was, so I had to drive down there last night to get it.

I had to remember where I last left it...over a year ago! Was it in my locker? No. Then I had to retrace my steps and remember how exactly things happened a year and a half ago when I got the bad news.

After Dr. Lin told me I had cancer, I left the office stunned, of course, but the first call I made was to work to tell them I wouldn't be in- for a while. Things happened so fast.

Then I realized it took a few months before I went back to Dana Point to visit. But by then I was in another frame of mind, focused only on beating cancer. And over the course of my treatment, I would make other visits but that mesh glove was the last thing on my mind. But there it was, over the sink, waiting for me.

I also went and did a little grocery shopping. I have to pack a lunch again! No more food trucks or chasing down the Kogi truck or Dos Chinos, my favorites.

My shift today is 11-8. It's a shift that allows me to go home if I need to without affecting the department.

Baby steps.

As I told my supervisor, the only major problem I have now is my feet; they're swollen from all the chemo I endured. It's a common side effect and only time will take care of it. I bought some compression socks to help. I did some research and there's really nothing my doctor can give me.

Being on my feet all day is going to be a challenge. Beating cancer was the ultimate challenge though. So going back to work?

Piece of cake.

First Day of Work – July 10, 2013 7:57 A.M.

I survived. It wasn't easy. But I'm glad it's over. Do I have to go back..? What was I thinking...

Actually, everything went well. If it wasn't for the condition of my feet (the swelling), it would have been a great day, but I have to deal with the fact that my feet are swollen and it will take some time for them to get better.

The day started out rather comically. I had bought new comfortable shoes and had to buy some new pants. My weight gain was on purpose. Going into 12 rounds of chemo I was very nervous. I felt if I gained a little weight it would help me get through the chemo, in case I started to experience diarrhea or a lot of nausea. I gained more than a little weight but it didn't bother me or my doctors.

I'm going to lose the weight – that I'm not worried about – so the pants were to accommodate my weight gain. I start to get dressed and go to put on my shirt and…oh, fuck! The shirt doesn't fit! Now I'm embarrassed.

I don't have enough time to go buy a bigger shirt so I call work and talk to Tim, the store manager and explain my predicament. Tim was the store manager at the Dana Point Gelson's during the strike and he is now in Newport. He said he had some shirts that would fit. Problem solved. Whew!

I start my shift and I will be helping out Don in the seafood department. Cool. Don, like me, used to work for Vons. He's very close to retirement. He's a pro and has probably forgotten more than I know. He starts showing me the new fish case and how they do things now. After about a half-hour my brain is ready to explode from information overload.

Ouch.

I used to do this, right? They say it's like riding a bike. Yeah! On the Tour de France! But by lunchtime I'm feeling OK. It was the last two hours of my shift that I got really tired and my feet were killing me. I was barely able to walk to my car. Dead man walking!

I feel fine this morning and I'm ready for another day at work. The day ended with some bad news – more like devastating.

My Dad has cancer again, now for the third time. He survived prostate and esophageal cancer. Now it's in his bladder and it's aggressive. I don't know much more. I was at work when I found out and now I'm trying to figure how I can go see him.

I have this damn job now.

Getting Back to Work, Getting Back to Normal – July 23, 2013 10:55 P.M.

Two weeks of work now and little by little, things are almost back to normal. I really needed this – to get back to a regular routine. And of course, getting a paycheck is pretty cool too.

It's been a challenge.

I love my job as a meat cutter because of both the mental aspect combined with the daily physical work. I have always treated cutting meat as an art, a lost art, if you will. Hopefully, I've been able to carry on this trade as it was meant to be. Like the tremendous support I experienced during my fight with cancer, the support at work has been awesome. I have big shoes to fill, my own. I set the bar pretty high and I'm almost there.

I saw my primary Doctor, Dr. Lin, last Friday. He looked at my feet, which are still swollen. He asked me why my oncologist wasn't as concerned about the condition of my feet. I told him with a shrug, "They're more concerned with killing my cancer, this side effect will go away, and they know that."

If I had a side effect that was really bothering me they would address it and do everything possible to help me. So Dr. Lin prescribed me a diuretic: a very small pill to help with the water retention. I only take half a pill daily and it's helping.

We also talked about my weight gain. Crazy, huh? I didn't lose my hair and I gained weight. Go figure. Chemo affects everyone differently.

I was not active for a year and a half and it caught up with me. But it's just another challenge and I'm up for it. Getting into shape is my priority. The chances of me getting another kind of cancer are now very good.

That's reality.

If it happens, I want to be physically ready for it.

And I will be.

The good news is the results from my blood work are good. Except for some elevated toxicity in my liver from the chemo, I am very healthy. My cholesterol is normal. Triglycerides? Normal . This tells me that my weight gain is temporary.

I thanked my brother Kevin, who has been doing a lot of the cooking for me throughout this journey. He has a garden with all kinds of veggies. He cooks chicken and ground turkey. He does eat red meat but doesn't cook it. That's what I do. So thanks to him I do get in some healthy meals. And my blood work showed that. Yay!

I Have No Health Benefits! WTF! – August 2, 2013 9:09 P.M

I have belonged to my Union since 1982. I've walked many a picket line. I've been a shop steward and a picket captain. I've paid my dues. Up until I had cancer, I've only had to use my health benefits for regular doctor visits. I'd never had an operation. I'd never had to be hospitalized. My cancer treatment started in January 2012, and by September 2012 I had to pay Cobra monthly $547.

I had apparently exhausted my benefits. And the only reason I found this out is because I called my union trust fund to make my premium payment, a modest $30 or $40, and they told me as of September I had to pay Cobra – this was on August 31, 2012.

I had Dr. appointments lined up for the whole month of September. I was still recovering from my surgery. Home Health nurses were visiting me three times a week.

But no one called me.

If I hadn't made that phone call I would still be fighting the tremendous bills I would have incurred.

I had no choice but to pay Cobra. I also didn't have the strength to go to the union and raise hell about my benefits and why I didn't receive a courtesy call to explain to me what was going on. All the strength that I had was focused on my healing. All the support that everyone was sending me on Twitter and Facebook, phone calls, texts – all that positive energy was how I was able to get through some very tough times.

Of course, considering all the medical attention I needed and the six months of chemo that I still had to endure, the Cobra payments were well worth it. Still...

After 30 years, you would think I would be given a little more than just eight months of coverage.

Which brings me to today: August 2, 2013. I've been working now for almost a month. When I made my Cobra payment for July I asked about paying for August. Did I qualify for insurance?

NO.

My benefits won't kick in until September so I would have to pay for August. I don't have any appointments for August. 'See you in three months' they told me in June, during that great, happy day when the results of my PET Scan came in. "No more cancer."

So I've been thinking that while I should pay for August, I can really use that $547 to pay some bills I've been holding off on. Hmm…I ran it by one of my co-workers and he said, "What if something happened? It's better to be safe with insurance than sorry without!"

Yeah, I thought…pay the Cobra, one more month.

"Hi! My name is Robert Flores and I would like to pay my Cobra."

"Okay, you're social ?"

"xxx-xx-xxxx."

"Okay, it looks like you have exhausted your Cobra benefits, sir."

"Whaaaaaaaaaaaaa!? I thought I had 18 months of Cobra?!"

"Yes, 18 months but if you collect workers comp or disability you only get 11 months."

"Well…I don't have any doctor appointments and I really didn't want to pay anyway."

"Just be careful and congratulations on beating cancer."

"Okay, thanks…"

Nice lady. Not her decision – just doing her job. But What. The. Fuck!!!

After all I've been through. I cannot believe this. What if I needed more treatment? What if my cancer had spread to my liver or lymph nodes? Does anyone give a fuck..?

I know you all care. You have had my back for the last year and a half. And now I have yours – each and every one of you. I sure didn't do this alone.

I'm just warming up.

I have the strength now.

The strength to find out why I have no benefits. Someone at my union better have the answers.

This is bullshit.

I Missed My Anniversary...Life Is Great! – August 17, 2013 9:35 P.M.

On July 26, 2012 I was in the operating room having my cancerous tumor and rectum removed. The operation, performed by Dr. Anita Gregory, saved my life. A year has passed and I'm back at work, so how will I commemorate this important day?

Should I celebrate?

Say a prayer ?

Call my Doctors and thank them?

Unfortunately, I did none of the above because the day passed and I totally forgot about all of it. It wasn't until July 29th that I realized that such a significant day had come and gone. In a lot of ways, this is a good thing.

While I will never, ever forget that day and the eight days I stayed in the hospital, my life is now, almost back to normal. Work has been great and I'm almost back to where I was before my diagnosis. I'm having fun at my job and I'm also spending time with friends and supporting them in their endeavors.

I attended a showing of pictures that my friend Art Meza takes of lowriders. It was in Highland Park at a store named Mi Vida. Also there that night were Donna, Alicia, Alondra and Deadlee who was escorting his Mom, Margaret. She was so sweet. It was a great turnout and I wish nothing but success for Art and his family.

On July 28 I attended a Dodger game with Paula Maez who was visiting from Arizona; it was the game where Puig hit the home run in the bottom of the 11th. Yes, we stayed until the end. Great times... normal times.

I still have not heard about my benefits, or rather, my lack of benefits. This upsets me. I won't let this die, one way or another, but I also want to concentrate on all the positive things in my life. I will deal with the union.

Getting back to normal doesn't mean I have forgotten about cancer.

Since my diagnosis, I have been on a website sponsored by the American Cancer Association. It's called 'What's Next.' I joined the site to hopefully find a mentor, someone, who like me, had the specific tumor that made my cancer "highly unusual." I never did find that mentor but I stayed on the site and I did learn a lot.

People post questions every day and if I am able to help I do. Now that I am a veteran of 18 chemo sessions, 28 radiation treatments, 26 Erbitux treatments and my surgery I have been able to answer some questions for the new members. It's very gratifying when someone says, "Thank you!"

Please follow on Twitter @AmateurChemist, aka Andrew Youssef. Andrew has Stage 4 colon cancer and he writes a column for the OC Weekly about his battle with it. He also photographs concerts for them and writes reviews. He's a great person and I'm proud to call him my friend. He's a badass cancer crusher but he can always use the support. He's going to fuck cancer just like I did!

I Also Have A Dream – August 28, 2013 10:02 A.M.

No, not that kind of dream. Sorry. During my year and a half of treatment I don't remember any dreams or even if I did dream. I might have been under too many drugs. I didn't start dreaming until my treatment ended. I was finally able to remember a few of those dreams.

This one dream in particular was a little weird and somewhat shocking. It was so startling in fact, that I posted about it on two separate cancer websites, asking if anyone with a permanent colostomy had ever had a similar dream. No one responded.

Maybe it touched a nerve. Maybe it was too personal. On these cancer websites it's pretty much anything goes so I was surprised at the lack of response.

Supposedly, your dreams can tell a lot about you or the subliminal you. I don't really know. It was a simple dream about a simple act - something that you do every day, probably at least twice a day. Something that I can't do anymore.

I must miss doing this simple act because I dreamt about it. I'm fine with the results of my treatment. It saved my life. I wish that I didn't have to have a colostomy but it's been the least of my worries. Really.

So after my dream I was wondering if there was anything wrong with me. Am I really happy? Am I, deep down, OK with things? I shrug and tell myself how lucky I am to be alive, to be back at work, to have the best friends anyone could have. I'm very honest, even with myself. If anyone else with a colostomy has had this dream, I'd like to know, if that's ok with you. I had a dream…I had dream that I pooped.

Follow up With Dr. Ash – September 9, 2013 9:55 A.M.

I had a follow up visit with my radiologist, Dr. Ash. It went well. Yay. His nurse, Rebecca, didn't recognize me without my beard and crazy hair. She was very complimentary on my clean look.

Dr. Ash told me to really concentrate on losing weight. More cardio! And I will. Yeah! Other than that. "See you in six months."

On my way to the parking structure, I ran into Jaime, my surgeon's nurse. She also was heavy on the compliments. Wow! I should wear this Raiders shirt more often!

I told her to please say hi to Dr. Gregory. I've wanted to write thank you notes to all my doctors. I should get on that.

Next stop, Dr. Lin, to see about my feet, which are still swollen.

One step – ouch – at a time.

Promoted – September 19, 2013 8:47 P.M.

Talk about a sweet comeback. Gelson's Supermarket, my employer, is opening a new store in Long Beach and I have been chosen to be part of the team there.

It's been two months now since I've been back to work. It was very tough at first, very. But now I'm almost 100-percent and by November, I will definitely be at 110.

The store will be in the Belmont Shore area of Long Beach on 2nd and PCH. I will be in charge of the Seafood department, the largest seafood case in the chain.

They expect the seafood department to be one of the focal points of the store. I can't wait. I received a very classy letter from a very classy company.

I especially like the commitment to excellence part. ;)

I Saw My Ancestors Last Night and They Were Me – October 13, 2013 3:33 P.M.

Last week, October 2nd, I attended a reading by Chicana punk rocker and author, Alice Bag, at my favorite library in Cypress Park. It was a great performance and I was able to visit with my good friends, Art Meza, his wife, Anna and their kids. My friends Donna and Alicia were also there and I met Monica, finally.

It just so happened, that Alice Bag was performing this week here in my hometown, of [9]SanTana at El Centro Cultural de Mexico. It turned out to be the best suggested donation of $10 I have ever spent! It was a full slate of performers who sang, rapped, danced and recited poetry with so much passion. It was hosted by Seeds of Resistance, a spiritual, autonomous, grassroots collective empowering [10]Womyn of all ages, through art.

To start the festivities, about six dancers dressed in Native Indian clothing came out. We were told the dances they were doing but I would have liked more information - it was so interesting and they danced well.

After about 45-minutes they brought out another Indian, native to Orange County, a Juaneno Indian. Her name was Michelle and she came out to bless the room and all of us. I am part Juaneno from my Dad's mother's side - my Grandma Petra. Michelle explained what she was doing as she burned incense. Michelle is 'Keeper of the Staff' of the Juaneno Indian Tribe and she brought the Staff to use to bless the room.

The Staff has traveled throughout the Western hemisphere being used in different ceremonies. I was riveted by this ceremony and memories of my Grandma Petra, my Tia Anita, Tio Juan, Uncle Pete and of someone I had never met, my great Grandmother Anastacia Majel. As soon as this part of the program was over I went up to Michelle and introduced myself.

"Hi, my name is Robert and I'm part Juaneno."

"Oh, hi, brother!" Michelle replied.

I told her that my great grandmother is Anastacia Majel, my family name is Flores and we're from the Logan neighborhood. That didn't

---

9   Chicano slang for Santa Ana, California.
10   Alternate spelling of "women" used by some feminists.

seem to ring any bells with Michelle but she let me hold the Staff and pose for a picture.

Michelle said, "Go ahead and say a prayer."

I told her that I'd been praying since I saw the staff!

I held that Staff with so much pride. At the same time I was also humbled and honored to touch something that one of my ancestors might have used in a ceremony so many years ago.

My great grandmother Anastacia was interviewed by John P. Harrington who worked for the Smithsonian as an ethnologist. She was fluent in the Juaneno language and he recorded her. Those recordings are used today to teach the Juaneno language.

During my battle with cancer, I had the support of so many of you and I will always be eternally grateful. Whether it was prayer or positive thoughts, I appreciated everything. I also prayed constantly, mostly to La Virgen de Guadalupe.

While I believe in science, I also have my faith. And I also would pray to my relatives that have passed on, like my Grandma Petra and Tia Anita. They used to babysit us when our parents would go out. I can still hear my Tia Anita's voice as she told us bedtime stories that were straight out of Heaven.

Some people call me a walking miracle, and if so then I would like to nominate my Grandma and Tia for sainthood. A day doesn't go by when I don't think about where I was a year ago. During October, in 2012, I still had cancer, I was carrying a wound vac and just had my Foley catheter replaced by a supra pubic tube so that my fistula in my urethra would heal.

And when all that would eventually heal, I was still facing six months of chemotherapy. I literally shudder when I think of what I endured.

How did I do that?

I read about people that give up, it's too much. I feel for them, it's not an easy decision. But what's the alternative? Yeah…death.

FUCK YOU, CANCER!

I'm one crazy Mexican-American Juaneno Indian!!

The Burning – October 17, 2013 7:01 P.M.

Silver sulfadiazine cream 1% is the ointment and Aquaphor was another cream I used, along with aloe vera. After the first week and a half, my Dr. asked me if I was using the aloe on my butt and I said no. He said you need to put that on every night and I was like…OK.

So that night I put it on and had no idea how hot to the touch my ass was! I never touch my butt so I had no idea the radiation was so intense. I used the aloe on my butt, the Aquaphor along my groin and the silver sulfadiazine in my crack of my butt. Every night and every day.

I'm just telling you this because it happened to me and I hope it doesn't happen to you. By the end of my radiation it was so painful to poop; I describe it as if lava was coming out of my ass. Extreme pain – the kind that makes grown men cry. Of course the end result is that I'm still here, alive and cancer free.

My anxiety was always high going into radiation. Along with prayer, sometimes I would smoke weed to calm me down. Being exposed like that along with being attached to a chemo pump 24/7 was pretty tough. And it seemed like it would take forever!

Also the machine broke down about six times. It would just stop. They finally reconfigured the sequence but still I was very concerned and told them about it. Their machine that was shooting lasers up my ass and it was breaking down! Was it safe? I didn't think so but they fixed it.

My radiation would last almost 15-minutes. My tumor was rather large.

Follow-up Oncology Visit – October 22, 2013 2:40 P.M.

I have a follow-up visit with my oncologist in a few minutes. No anxiety. I just hope I don't get too emotional. They only saved my life. Happy tears. :-)

Happy Thanksgiving – November 28, 2013 8:44 A.M.

For me, every day is a day of thanks and giving. A year ago today,

I still had cancer. I was still recovering from my surgery. I was getting ready to do six months of chemo. Not a day goes by that I don't remind myself of this, especially if I'm having a rough day at work.

The fact that I'm at work is something to be very thankful for. I'm back at almost 100-percent productive – back to where I was before I got sick. Yay!

I'm getting ready to start prepping the turkey, chopping the veggies, making some breakfast and watching a lot of football! Enjoy your Thanksgiving Day but enjoy every day and thank you for your continued support!

Fuck cancer.

Where's the Complaint Department? – November 30, 2013 5:52 P.M.

I've had it up to here with this asshole called "Cancer." I hate this coward, Cancer. Picking on little kids…what a jerk. Who do I complain to?! Do I complain to the Man upstairs? Or should I complain to the Man downstairs? Is the Lady of the House in? There has to be someone in charge?

Every day, someone dies of cancer, someone is diagnosed with cancer or someone is going through treatment for cancer. Brilliant doctors and scientist are finding new ways to fight cancer. They're making progress but as far as a cure, I don't see one in the immediate future. So I want to complain. People complain about stuff all the time.

My steak was tough!

[Okay here's another one and it's free!]

It's cold in here!

[I'm sorry, let me turn up the heat.]

My turn…

I'm sick and tired of cancer getting people sick and I am really tired of people dying from cancer. Really, really fucking tired of this!

Is anyone listening?? HelllllllllllOOOOOOO. I'm talking to YOU!

Don't ignore me! I'm not leaving until YOU do something about this scumbag, Cancer.

Cancer is not welcome here and yet it always seems to just show up, unannounced and definitely uninvited. I'll even meet YOU halfway. I already kicked Cancer's ass. I fucked Cancer. Now I'm ready to completely eradicate it. Forever!

I hate cancer and I won't stop until cancer no longer exists. No more sick kids. No more sick friends and family.

No. More. Death.

My name is Robert and I fuck Cancer.

Shit – December 9, 2013 8:42 P.M.

Don't you just hate when you put on a new colostomy bag and it gets all shitty?

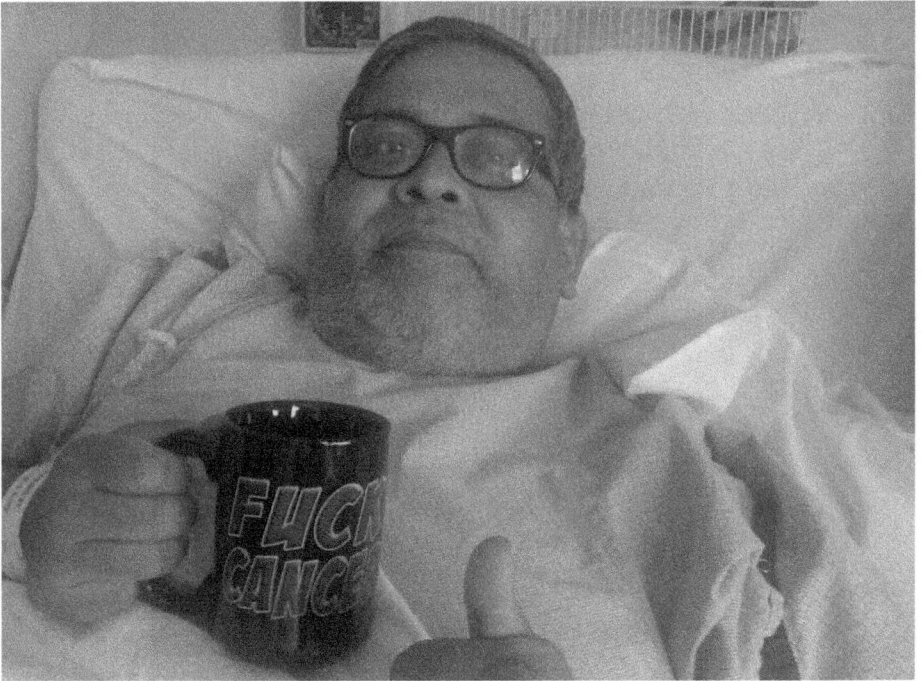

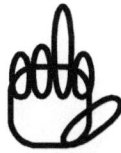

Part VI: ¡Fuck Cancer!

Don't Count the Days, Make the Days Count – December 10, 2013 7:12 P.M.

These are the words my dad said when he was told last week that he had six months to live. They are so much like the words of my friend Andrew Youseff who recently passed away from stage 4 colon cancer. Andrew told me he was "going to go down swinging." And he sure did!

Actually, I would say Andrew went down "rocking!" Andrew was a concert photographer and even in the last few weeks of his life, he was still at it. Depeche Mode was his last concert and two weeks later Andrew was gone. But he will never be forgotten. Rest in peace, my good friend.

I was lucky to meet Andrew, thanks to Gustavo Arellano, who introduced us earlier this year while I was going through chemo to fight my cancer (also stage 4 colon cancer). We all met at Memphis in Downtown SanTana.

Andrew took concert pictures for the OC Weekly where Gustavo is the Editor in Chief, or as we all call him the Mexican in Chief. Ha! We talked about chemo and traded colostomy stories. It was great to finally meet someone who I could ask cancer questions. Andrew had all the answers.

He was already two years into his battle with cancer. He had already endured over 100 chemo treatments. Yes, 100.

I would eventually do a total of 18 treatments, no picnic for sure but 100 sounds almost impossible. But nothing was impossible with Andrew.

In addition to being a photog, he also had a day job working at the pharmacy at Long Beach Memorial. But taking concert photos was his passion. He never missed a deadline according to Gustavo. In fact, Andrew was so reliable that Gustavo didn't know about Andrew's condition for quite some time.

Andrew was a great mentor and inspiration, not only to me but to many others who read his blog (amateurchemist.tumblr.com), which became a weekly feature in the OC Weekly. Andrew made every day count.

In July, I went back to work after a year and a half of chemo, radiation, surgery and more chemo. In June, I was scanned and declared cancer free. At the same time my dad was diagnosed with bladder cancer.

This is my dad's third dance with cancer. He beat prostate and esophageal cancer. So he knew what he was in for and was very upbeat. They caught the cancer early and he wasn't in any pain. He started with chemo and I felt bad because now that I was working again I couldn't go and visit him but he kept me updated and everything seemed to be going as planned.

About two months ago we were talking and my dad kept coughing. I asked him if he was sick and he said no, he only coughed in the morning and it would go away. I was skeptical because it sounded like bronchitis and I knew that since he was going through chemo, getting sick with a weakened immune system was the last thing he needed. I told him to at least put on a sweater.

He started to have a few complications with his kidneys and unbeknownst to me, he was losing his appetite.

The week before Thanksgiving he was in the hospital for what they thought was pneumonia. Great. I was getting over a slight case of bronchitis myself so I waited a few days before I went to see him.

I walked into the room and was shocked to see his condition. He looked terrible – thin and fatigued and somewhat incoherent.

It wasn't pneumonia; the cancer had spread to his lung.

Deep breath…

Fuck cancer! Fuck cancer! Fuck cancer! Fuck cancer! Fuck cancer! Fuck cancer! Fuck cancer! Fuck cancer! Fuck cancer! Fuck cancer! Fuck cancer! Fuck cancer! Fuck cancer! Fuck cancer! Fuck cancer! Fuck cancer! Fuck cancer! Fuck cancer!

Fuck cancer! Fuck cancer! Fuck cancer! Fuck cancer! Fuck cancer! Fuck cancer!
Fuck cancer! Fuck cancer! Fuck cancer! Fuck cancer! Fuck cancer! Fuck cancer!
Fuck cancer! Fuck cancer! Fuck cancer! Fuck cancer! Fuck cancer! Fuck cancer!
Fuck cancer! Fuck cancer! Fuck cancer! Fuck cancer! Fuck cancer! Fuck cancer!
Fuck cancer! Fuck cancer! Fuck cancer! Fuck cancer! Fuck cancer! Fuck cancer!
Fuck cancer! Fuck cancer! Fuck cancer! Fuck cancer! Fuck cancer! Fuck cancer!
Fuck cancer! Fuck cancer! Fuck cancer! Fuck cancer! Fuck cancer! Fuck cancer!
Fuck cancer! Fuck cancer! Fuck cancer! Fuck cancer! Fuck cancer! Fuck cancer!
Fuck cancer! Fuck cancer! Fuck cancer! Fuck cancer! Fuck cancer! Fuck cancer!
Fuck cancer! Fuck cancer! Fuck cancer! Fuck cancer! Fuck cancer! Fuck cancer!
Fuck cancer! Fuck cancer! Fuck cancer! Fuck cancer! Fuck cancer! Fuck cancer!
Fuck cancer! Fuck cancer! Fuck cancer! Fuck cancer! Fuck cancer! Fuck cancer!
Fuck cancer! Fuck cancer! Fuck cancer! Fuck cancer! Fuck cancer! Fuck cancer!

I stayed the rest of the day. He was being discharged and I wanted to help. He could barely walk. The next day he had an appointment with his oncologist. I had the day off and I had a walker at home. I went home with it when I left the hospital after my surgery. I knew he would need it now.

So I met him and his wife, Sylvia, and helped him get out of the car (they brought a wheelchair). Sylvia asked if I wanted to go into the meeting but I thought it would be better if I stayed outside and waited.

Nothing really happened, the doctor told him to go home and get some rest that he would start chemo after Thanksgiving on December 2nd.

The day after Thanksgiving Sylvia had to take him back to the hospital because he was having trouble breathing. On Saturday morning Andrew Youseff passed away, after an almost three-year battle with colon cancer and now the cancer is in both of my dad's lungs. It's very aggressive.

No fucking shit.

I go see him on Sunday and he actually looks good. He's eating, thanks to the marijuana laced candy my brother, Chito, is giving him. Yeah. It surely won't hurt but all his doctors are on holiday, so we won't know anything until Monday.

Monday comes and nothing. They need to do more tests.

By Thursday, they finally tell the family that there's nothing they can do. It's a rare form of cancer that has already damaged his kidneys and lungs to where even chemo won't help.

But my Dad's a fighter. He's already kicked cancer's ass twice.

He's a lucky man and at almost 80, still has a lot to live for. He says he doesn't want to die. That's all I needed to hear. Whatever you want Dad. We're all here and we're all going to fight with you. We're looking at alternative and holistic methods.

It's so true that old saying: The apple doesn't fall far from the tree.

I'm looking at the tree and I'm in awe of its strength, its wisdom and I know that it's too soon for this tree to fall.

December 12th, 2013: My Two Year Cancerversary – December 12, 2013 6:09 P.M.

I'm not celebrating. No, nothing like that but I am thankful. I'm very thankful on this day, which is also the day we honor La Virgen De Guadalupe. I mentioned it this morning to my boss, Mark, who coincidently was my boss in 2011 when I got the bad news.

We were at the Gelson's in Dana Point and now we are in the new Gelson's in Long Beach. He remembers that day well, and the phone call.

"I won't be able to work tomorrow…or for a while. I have cancer."

Even saying those words now seems surreal.

I have cancer…

And that's all I knew. I didn't know it would take a year and a half to get better. I thought I would be out for six-months. Really. Not even close!

But here I am two years later, back at work and doing well. And as my friend Paula says, "Still kicking cancer's ass!"

Hell Yes!

I am very thankful to all the support everyone has given me these last two years. I could not have survived the chemo, the radiation, the surgery and the additional chemo without YOU!

My friends and family are the Best! What's really been great is meeting everyone these last couple of years. We've had some good times and I look forward to many more. There are still a few people I haven't met yet but I know I will.

My journey has been full of tough times, I did have some complications after my surgery but I healed. All my follow ups with my doctors have been good – real good. But my journey with cancer isn't over and I don't expect it to be.

I'm here writing this blog in the hopes that I can reach out to those with cancer. If I can be of any help, answer questions, or just be there for you, you can count on me. I'll listen to your story because I believe it's important that you tell it.

I'll listen to you cry because we all cry. It's ok to cry but mostly I will always be here to help you kick cancer's ass! Fuck cancer!

Dad – December 17, 2013 12:22 P.M.

Hail Mary, full of grace, my dad is dying. Hail Mary, full of grace, I need a favor...

Hail Mary, full of grace, I'm standing here watching my dad die. Cancer is slowly killing him. He's fighting.

He looks at me.

I smile.

I refuse to cry. Not now. It's hard for him to swallow so he's dehydrating. He's cramping. He's not eating. He coughs.

And coughs... I hold his hand. He says he's OK. But He's not.

I'm praying.

When in doubt, pray...

Hail Mary, full of grace, fuck cancer.

Talking Shit, with your host Robert the Bold – December 18, 2013 3:09 P.M.

The other day at work, two of my coworkers went to the restroom at the same time. That left me and the boss, Mark.

I said "Are those two going to go shit at the same time?"

Mark shakes his head and says, "I just hope they're not using the same stall."

So I tell Mark, "You know, if your crew all had colostomies you wouldn't have this problem."

He laughed. "You're right, Robert. You're right."

I never miss an opportunity to make having a colostomy a positive thing. That's how I survive. Every day.

It's better than having a pity party, which I understand some people with a colostomy seem to have. We all deal with this our own way and this is one example of how I can spin this thing.

Please feel free to share some of your shittiest stories here on 'Talking Shit, with your Host, Robert The Bold.' :)

Dad: I Love You – December 19, 2013 6:04 P.M.

After my last visit with my dad on Tuesday, the nurse showed up and immediately called 911 to get him to the nearest ER. He was severely dehydrated. He's home now.

Earlier today my sister, Denise, called me to tell me he only had a few hours left. I left work, picked up my brother, Kevin, and here we sit.

Soon he'll be with his mom and dad and his brothers, Eddie and Alonzo. He won't be suffering.

My Dad is the oldest of five brothers and one sister. He grew up on Logan Street in Santa Ana. He attended Santa Ana High School.

Bob Flores. Everyone calls him Bob.

He's a fighter but the fight is over. He didn't lose. Nope. He's a winner in my book.

I love you Dad.

Holy Mary Mother of God Pray For Us Sinners Now and at the Hour of Death, Amen – December 19, 2013 10:43 P.M.

My Dad has six children. I was thinking how at each birth, he impatiently waited and waited for our arrival; the proud new papa pacing in the waiting room. He was happy that we were all healthy babies and now here we are, his progeny, waiting and praying for his death – a death that will end his suffering.

The suffering I saw firsthand, on Tuesday. Having recently survived cancer, I know how evil it can be. What I endured was nothing compared to what my dad has just gone through. And He never complained. Never.

I saw him continue to fight the cancer as it was aggressively killing him. No man, woman or child should have to suffer like this, but Cancer could not care less who it kills. The coward's coward.

My dad's blood pressure is slowly going down but his heart is strong. The nurse says he could literally have no blood pressure and his heart will continue to pump.

The heart of a lion has no master. Fuck you, Cancer!

Passing – December 20, 2013 3:24 P.M.

My dad, Bob Flores, is an angel. He passed a few moments ago. No more suffering. Fuck cancer.

Thank you everyone for your prayers and support.

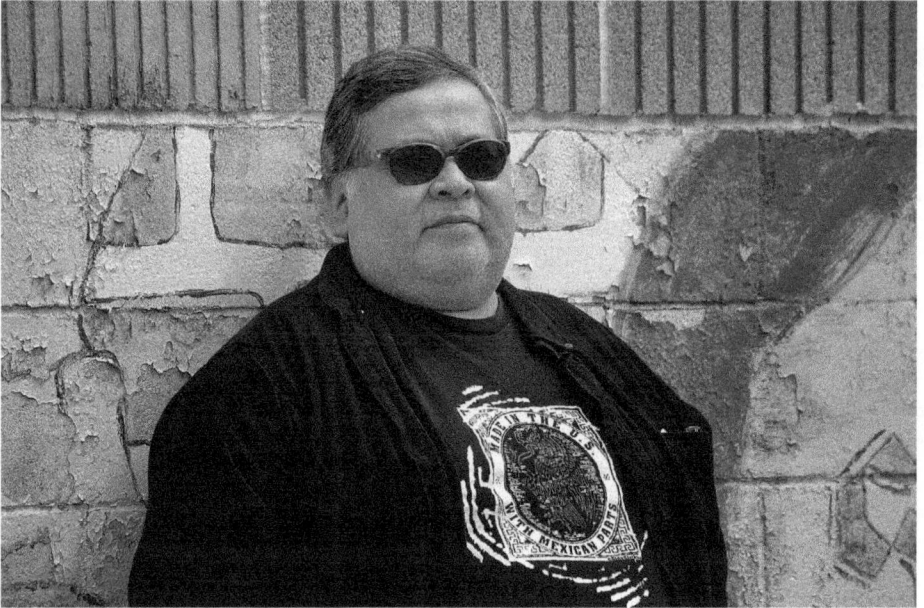

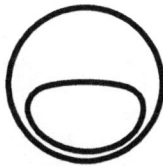

Part VII: Gravity

Memories of an Ex-Farter – January 29, 2014 9:09 P.M.

Farting isn't fun but it is funny. Farting is a natural bodily function. The first fart was probably followed by the first laugh. They call the dog man's best friend because Fido has taken the blame for many a fart.

Farting starts in your gut, then travels through your intestines and comes out your bum. But not for me.

I don't have a rectum so it comes out my stoma and into my colostomy bag. It sort of sounds like a fart but there's no signature stink. My colostomy bag has a filter to keep everything smelling like a rose. Ha! I can't fart anymore but I can sure make you laugh, without all the aroma.

This weekend is Super Bowl Sunday. Yay! I'm going to Vegas with my brother, Kevin. I haven't worked on Super Bowl Sunday for about 26 years. I was in New York in 1987 when the Giants beat the Broncos. They played here at the Rose Bowl but I was in Manhattan. I even went to the celebration in Giants Stadium when the team came back.

I was in Vegas last year for the Super Bowl when I was in the middle of 12 chemo sessions. I still had a great time. I always have a good time with my brothers. I didn't drink but maybe two beers during the game. But I was there and bet on the Ravens. Winner!

During my year and a half treatment for cancer, cancer took over my life but I didn't allow it to control my life. If you're going through treatment now for cancer, OWN IT! Take charge of your treatment. Do your homework. Ask questions. Challenge your doctors! You won't be hurting their feelings. Don't worry about them. Worry about yourself.

Find a support group, whether it's on-line or in person. Talk to someone who has been through this Hell. That will save your life.

It's hard to find any normalcy in your life but by going to Vegas for Super Bowl weekend I was able to tell cancer, "Fuck you!"

I couldn't do a lot of things that I would normally do but to do something that I had been doing for a long time was very special, especially with Kevin.

Not only did he cook many of my meals for me but he picked me up after every chemo session, 18 in all. He picked up my medicine when I wasn't able to go. He would take me to the doctor when I couldn't drive myself. No complaints. He'll never pay for a drink this weekend.

It's my turn. I got this.

World Cancer Day – February 4, 2014 10:45 A.M.

Hmm…World Cancer Day. Not exactly a Hallmark Holiday. For me, even though I'm at the moment, cancer free, and every day is World Cancer Day.

Until there is a cure and no one has to suffer from this cowardly disease, I will not rest easy. Every day I am thankful for my health, for my family and friends. Every day I try to reach out to someone, anyone, with cancer. If I can help, I surely will. So today, I will re-post some of my stories in the hope that it might help. It is a reminder of what it took me to get through all my treatment and especially how everyone was so instrumental in getting me through it.

Sometimes – February 16, 2014 8:50 P.M.

Sometimes I'm reminded that I have a colostomy bag attached to my body and think: OH, SHIT!

Then I snap out of it and say, "Fuck you, Cancer! I'm alive!"

Cold Beer – February 17, 2014 8:02 P.M.

I'm going to put on some very warm clothes and go drink some very cold beer…Who's with Me?

Lucky – February 21, 2014 12:19 P.M.

Everyday is My lucky Day!

Dixie – March 1, 2014 5:20 A.M.

My stoma is so clean you can whistle Dixie with it…

Gravity – March 1, 2014 10:48 P.M.

I just watched the movie Gravity for the second time. It might or might not be the movie of the year but for me it did have the message of the year. And like the first time I watched it, the message was the same: NEVER GIVE UP!

It is a beautiful movie to watch. The constant background is from space and as all the action takes place you're watching earth in all its outer space beauty. I also liked both Sandra Bullock and George Clooney – very simple in the way of dialogue.

I'm sure other movies have been made with the same message. But because this one is so recent and since I'm still and will always be overwhelmed by what I went through with cancer, it really struck home with me. NEVER GIVE UP!

For a lot of us, it's life or death. Cancer doesn't fuck around. To survive cancer means to go through rigorous and torturous treatment. And sadly, some people do give up. But I can't pass judgment, no way.

I don't agree with it but to make that decision, to stop treatment, can't be easy. We all have our limits. But my will to live was stronger than any chemo, radiation, surgery, complications from surgery and so on.

A year ago today, I was still going through chemo plus the additional Erbitux. My life was just one treatment after another; waiting for the results of another round of blood tests and the occasional blood transfusion because I was so anemic.

A lot of you are going through all these various treatments right now. And I know how you feel. I know it seems like there is no end to all this. When can I get off this roller coaster!?

It will end. It did for me and it will for you. And hopefully you'll be giving sage advice to the newbies; the ins and outs, the ups and downs.

When you do get that chance to help those who unfortunately follow in our footsteps, tell them to NEVER GIVE UP.

And also tell them: FUCK CANCER!

Tacos, Bobbleheads and Cancer, Oh My! – April 3, 2014 8:34 P.M.

What a great couple of days off I just had, and I needed them. It all started on Tuesday evening; I had to work 10 –7 that day and I was tired when I got home. I decided to go have a couple of beers at Noble Ale Works and also hoped that there would be a food truck there. The Angels were playing and it was Mike Trout bobblehead night.

I got there about 8:30 p.m. and bummer, no food truck. Well, I'll just have a couple of beers and head out to a delicious dinner of Del Taco later. Noble is arguably the best brewery in OC, in my humble opinion, and they always have something new brewing. I was enjoying their latest brew, Simcoe Showers, when the Angel fans, with their Trout bobbleheads in hand, started to show up.

The game wasn't over but the Angels were losing so it was beer o'clock. A nice couple came in, ordered their beers and sat down at the long table I was sitting at. I asked them, "Where's your bobbleheads?"

They smiled, "In the car!"

So we talked about how bad the Angels already looked in only the second game of the season and we agreed on how good the beer was at Noble. Great minds think alike, or so they say. I finished my second beer and was about to leave. I said goodbye to my new friends and thanked them for the conversation. The young man, Jerry, said, "Wait I have something for you."

We walked out to his car and he told me, "We want you to have our extra Mike Trout bobblehead. We have two and only need one."

"Really? Wow. Thank you so much," I told Jerry, "Hope to see you two again and I'll buy the next round."

Amazing.

The next day, I was to meet up with Art Meza, his wife Anna and David Cid in Echo Park, at Guisados. It was my first time here and let me tell you, it was great; fresh corn tortillas, chicken, beef and pork tacos, all with a variety of sauces and chiles. They also have shrimp and chicharron ones. They have the usual horchata and jamaica drinks but I had the melon, fresh agua de cantaloupe. The best!

Guisados was letting Art show his photography and one wall was dedicated to his work. I'm sure Art will sell many of his pictures of lowriders and different views of the City of Angels. Great friends and good comida!

I then headed to Montebello to catch the movie Cesar Chavez. I wanted to see it with gente. I ended up in Pico Rivera and caught a matinee. I enjoyed the movie. It wasn't perfect but it's about time someone made a movie of this great man.

After the movie (and coming out of my taco coma), I went to Willowick golf course to hit a bucket of balls. I haven't been able to play golf for the last two years (too busy kicking cancer's ass), but I won't miss the Cinco de Mayo Tournament this year!

I walk up to buy a bucket of balls and the golf pro, Kenny, says, "Hi Robert!"

Really? I haven't played in two years but Kenny remembers me. Wow. Amazing!

Today, I also had a follow up with my oncologist. I actually missed my appointment last month. These follow ups are every three months now and unless someone reminds me, well, I forget stuff.

Work has been hell and I'm still trying to get some normalcy in my life. Time really does fly by but these visits are necessary. I have been feeling fatigued lately.

During my treatment, I was extremely anemic, even needing two blood transfusions and countless shots to boost my hemoglobin. I made the appointment with Esther the PA because it's too hard to see Dr. Mahmood and if you do get in he makes you wait for hours, he's that busy.

Everyone was happy to see me. Long time no see Robert! I know, I know. I mentioned to the front desk that I also wanted to pay off my balance. She said she'd look into it. The nurse, Lourdes, drew some blood and they got the results right away.

Esther came in and went over everything. Looking Good! But still anemic.

She prescribed a series of B12 shots, which I took to two different pharmacies with no luck. I called the office and they will find a pharmacy that stocks the B12 and send it to my house. Bam!

Esther also said I was due for a PET Scan so she will get that approved. Other than that, see you in three months!

When I was walking out, the girl at the front desk told me I didn't have a balance. I told her I thought I owed $300. She said, "No, you're good."

Really? Wow. Amazing! Fuck cancer. :)

Haha! – April 3rd, 2014 8:17 A.M.

Haha! I just farted in my face! Which is entirely possible when you have a stoma. I was changing my bag and cleaning my stoma when I ripped one.

So Funny.

It's not the first time and won't be the last. Have a nice day!

Great News! – April 23, 2014 3:15 P.M.

But first, the sort of bad news…I'm still fat. And very anemic. But I am working on it! It ain't easy but nothing worth it is.

Back to the great news.

Last week, I had a PET Scan. This was my third one. The first one was in January of 2012 and it showed where all the cancer was. The second one was last year in June, and that one showed zero cancer. This last one also came back negative for cancer. Yay!

It has been almost a whole year cancer free – what a relief. There is a certain amount of anxiety when we take these tests. I try not to let it show but it is there. I say "we" because I'm not alone. I've met so many that have gone through cancer treatment and so many that are still going through it. I follow them on social media and will continue to follow and support them.

I never want myself or anyone to go through what I went through again. Unfortunately, the odds are that I will, but I don't live in fear. I live every day to its fullest. Yesterday was a prime example.

I took my brother Kevin to the Dodger game, it was blanket night. Before the game, we ate tacos at Guisados, enjoyed a couple of Dodger Dogs during the game, then went to Original Tommy's for a chili burger.

These are the best days of my life.

These tests, PET Scans and CBC bloodwork will always be part of my life. They are necessary to ensure that cancer doesn't come back... but if it does come back. Well, I guess I'll just have to kick its ass again!

Fuck you, Cancer!

I Don't Sweat the Small Stuff...But Still – May 1, 2014 8:34 A.M.

Surviving Cancer 101

One day at a time. Sounds simple enough, right? Follow ups, exercise, diet...and dealing with ignorance.

I've been back at work now for nine months. It's been hard. Physically and mentally it's been a challenge. Being extremely anemic hasn't helped. I don't think it's affected my work. My numbers are good. Solid. My department head gave me a very good yearly review and primarily, my production is above average. I work hard. It's called work ethic.

The other day the supervisor comes in, nice guy, has always supported me. First he talks to the department head and his assistant. Then he takes me out back to talk to me – kind of a pep talk. Nothing negative. He never said I was doing anything wrong or they were unhappy with me. His message was basically, "We need you to work harder, go the extra mile. Be a leader," so on and so forth. Then he played the C-card.

He actually went there.

We were there for you Robert. We stood up for you and supported you...

I can't believe he's saying this. Of course I know that they kept my job for a year and a half. Of course I'm grateful. I've written about it here on my blog how lucky I am to work for this company. How my union told me that no other company would have kept my job for that long. They only have to keep it for six months then either you come back or they can legally fire you. I never gave the details on how they made this happen because I didn't know if what they did was legal and I didn't want to get certain people in trouble.

Keeping my job for the time I was going through treatment was a blessing. It eliminated a ton of stress that I didn't need to have. The stress of losing my job would have sent me into who knows how deep of a depression, and at a time when I needed to just concentrate on beating cancer. I'll always be grateful and I show it by working my ass off. I don't need to be reminded.

In all fairness I know this guy pretty well and recognized he was just the messenger. He was told by his boss to come in to talk to all of us. The company is not happy with the sales but I won't go into that.

Being diagnosed with cancer must be like opening the ultimate Pandora 's Box. What follows is different for everyone. It's a long road with so many ups and downs.

So fuck cancer and fuck ignorance too.

Cinco De Mayo Golf Tournament 2014 – May 4, 2014 7:29 A.M.

Over 25 years ago, four friends got together on Cinco de Mayo and played golf. The next year it was eight friends, then twelve and today there will be over 60 friends and relatives playing golf.

My longtime friend, Frank Martinez and his Dad, Mr. Martinez, have been running the tournament. They used to have it at golf courses all over Orange County and then Inland Empire but for the last ten years or so we have played at Willowick Golf Course in Santa Ana.

For $65 you get to play 18 holes and you get a nice lunch after the front nine. There are cash prizes and an all-you-can-eat, carne asada dinner, afterward. The Martinez family would host the after party for years, with Mrs. Martinez working hard on the side dishes and decorating their backyard, but now we have the awards and dinner there at Willowick. It makes it easier for everyone, especially Mrs. Martinez.

While the Masters Tournament in Augusta will award the winner with the coveted green jacket, we have something even more especial, the coveted Brown Jacket. We found it at a thrift store and I think the $1.95 tag is still on it. My comadre, Patty, sewed a custom patch for it. Forget the money; the Brown Jacket is the real prize. This year's winner will be able to wear it for the whole year; to the Sizzler, to Walmart, in the privacy of their home…wink-wink.

I haven't been able to play for the last two years. I had the PICC line in my left arm for a year and a half and two years ago I was also connected to a chemo pump 24/7. So today is a big day for me.

I am not a very good golfer nor do I claim to be but when I tee off I will consider myself a winner. I'll get teased for my horrific swing but that will be OK. I'll be surrounded by my friends and family who supported me throughout my journey with cancer. Every year I would show up to say hi to everyone. To let them know that I was doing well; that I was going to beat this cancer.

So, be warned, I will fill my timeline today with selfies…of my golf buddies; selfies of normalcy, of good times. Of life!

I might not ever win the Brown Jacket and wear it to In-N-Out but today is another step in healing and in winning the bigger prize. Gracias a Dios.

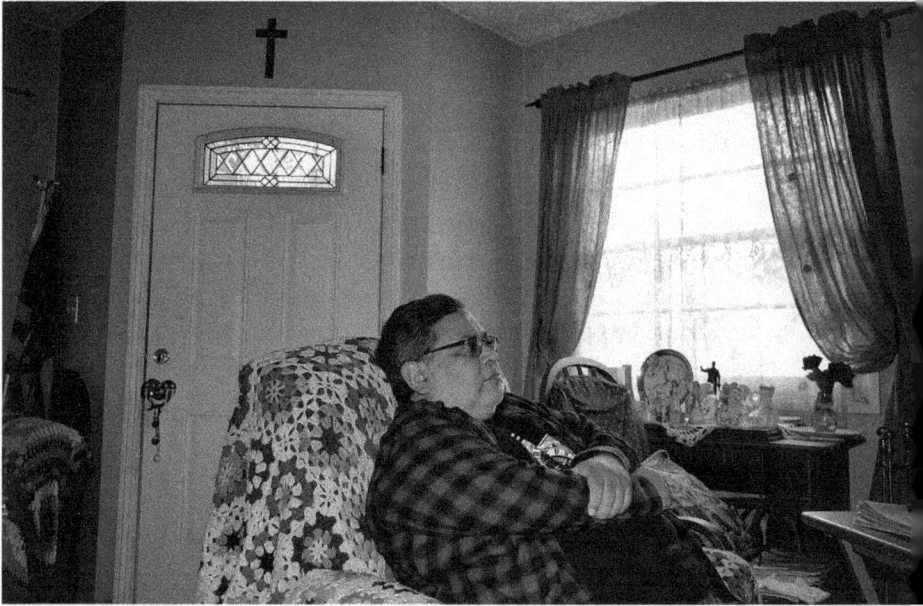

Part VIII: The Aftermath

Ed. Note: These entries are not dated but were written as afterthoughts and reflections by Robert.

What is Survivor's Guilt? Do I Have it?

L
ike a lot of people, today's news of baseball great Tony Gwynn's passing came as quite a shock. Even though we all knew he had been battling cancer for the last four years, he kept it very private and I don't blame him. Even after reading his son's, Tony Gwynn Jr., interview, that appeared in the Philadelphia Sunday paper, he didn't really give any indication about how ill his Dad really was. He did ask for prayers and acknowledged that Tony Sr. was really fighting his cancer. The article and interview was really about Father's Day and how he was going to celebrate it.

Did I know Tony Gwynn? No. But I really enjoyed watching him play for the Padres. He was one of the premier hitters of his generation, and I guess mine too. We were about the same age and I just turned 55. He was 54. Tony could have played anywhere else and made five times the money but he was loyal, not only to the Padres, but to the city of San Diego – a rare breed akin to the Angel's Jered Weaver, who has also decided to take less money to stay here in Anaheim.

A star on the field as well as off, Tony Gwynn was known as Mr. Padre. Of all the stats that Mr. Gwynn has accomplished, the one that stood out to me was the one with over 10,000 at bats. In his career, Tony Gwynn struck out a total of 434 times. Total! That's just incredible.

Anytime someone dies of cancer, it just pisses me off. Then I get sad, especially if it's a child. And then I think how lucky I am to be here.

Every cancer patient endures so much treatment and we all hope for the same outcome; to live. We all want to wake up another day and enjoy our family and friends. And while the percentage of survivors grows every day, it's still a small number compared to those who have not survived. Many do survive and go into remission, only to have the cancer come back. And when the cancer comes back, it comes back with a vengeance. The patient is still weak from all the treatment and the cancer is stronger and immune to the drugs from the previous treatments.

The news of Tony Gwynn's death, was at first, a shock, then rage, and now I'm a little scared. If this intelligent, accomplished athlete couldn't beat cancer, what are my chances? Really…Yes, I'm cancer free. But for how long?

Last year, my friend, Andrew, died of colon cancer in November, and then a month later I watched my Dad lose his life to cancer. But I don't feel guilty for surviving – for being alive.

I do feel something, though.

It's this overwhelming feeling of wanting to help, to listen. I've been there! I know what you're going through or what you might have to go through. Maybe it's not survivor's guilt but a sense of helplessness that I go through.

If I'm guilty of anything, it's not being able to do more.

Support Groups, the Internet and Tijuana

The support I received during this journey was tremendous. It came from family, friends and friends of friends. Plus, I met many new friends and supporters along the way. There were so many people willing to help.

Getting a ride to chemo, getting picked up from chemo, phone calls, texts and tweets from friends asking how I was doing – nothing but love. But even still, I wanted to talk to someone, like me, who had the exact cancer that I had. Someone that had already experienced this hell I was going through. Someone to tell me, "Hey, look, I survived and so will you, buddy."

Words alone cannot really describe what I was going through. I was looking for answers that only another person with colorectal cancer

AND the "highly unusual" tumor I had (that was "embedded in my pelvis" as Dr. Gregory put it), could give me. And I asked Dr. Gregory if she had another patient with the similar tumor. She said that my case was only the second time she had ever seen a tumor come out through the skin. Usually the tumor will go right up into the internal organs, the liver being the most common. So I went on-line.

Beware the internet! So scary. So dangerous. Well, I embraced the internet. I compare the internet to that wonderful city across the border, Tijuana! Great city! Crazy city.

If you're looking for trouble you'll find it. If you want to have fun or go shopping it's there. Pretty girls? They're there too. Drugs? What kind you want! In other words, it's up to you. Be responsible and own up to your actions. Don't blame the internet for your failed marriage or for your porn addiction. Go to Tijuana.

I found a site called WhatNext.com . It's affiliated with the American Cancer Association. You fill out a bunch of questions concerning your particular cancer and then it matches you up with other cancer patients. Not exactly Match.com but even though I never found a mentor I learned a lot from it and I'm currently still on the site.

Basically, the site is there for you to ask questions and since I was in the pool with other colorectal patients I was able to go to the forum and if I had a question there was always someone there to answer. As I earned my cancer-cred, I was also able to answer questions.

Every day, I receive an e-mail from the site with updates, new patients, and new questions and things like if I can answer a newbie's question. I try to give them my best answer from my experience.

Another internet option for me was Twitter. When I first signed up for Twitter, I thought it was only good for following food trucks and porn stars. Well, I still follow the food trucks. If you are not on Twitter, the way I like to describe it is, it's like texting but everyone that follows you can see it. For me, it started out as just something fun to do, shoot the breeze about sports or politics with people etc.

I do have to give major credit to a very good friend that I met on Twitter, yes, one of the very cool outcomes of Twitter is when you meet someone that you follow or that follows you. His name is Art Meza. He's a librarian in Los Angeles at the Cypress Park Library.

Seven Degrees of Art Meza! After the food trucks and porn stars,

I started to follow the Chicano cartoonist Lalo Alcaraz. Besides being funny and on point, we shared similar views politically and he was very accessible on Twitter. Then, I followed Gustavo Arellano, someone who I only knew through his columns in the OC Weekly; Ask a Mexican and The Hole in The Wall column where he would give insight on so many cool places to eat.

Then, what Twitter does, is suggest other people that are similar to those that you already follow. That's how I came to follow Art and he followed me. I also started to follow a fellow named Santino Rivera, poet, indie publisher and devoted Denver Bronco fan.

Prior to my cancer diagnosis, Santino and I would go back and forth with our rival football teams, I am a Raider fan. When Santino found out I had cancer, he asked me for my address and sent me two of his books of poetry. I took those books with me to my chemo treatments and discovered poetry.

As a kid I never really liked pizza here in the OC where I grew up. My first visit to New York City was in the early 80's and I was about 23-years-old. When I bit into that New York pizza, I realized what pizza was supposed to taste like. That's how I felt about Santino's poetry. So this is what poetry is supposed to taste like. This is how I talked. This is how I think.

Finally, during my chemo and radiation treatments, Art started to host book readings and poetry readings at his library branch. One of the first authors he had was Lalo Alcaraz, so I mustered up my strength and drove up to L.A. to meet this very funny and talented man whom, every day through his strip, La Cucaracha, would bring a smile to my face as I faced another day of treatment.

A few months later Art had Gustavo Arellano for a reading and there I was, somehow, able to meet another Twitter carnal. By then, I had other followers who were supporting me and I was able to meet them also, there at the Cypress Park library. I met Alicia, Emilio, Deadlee and eventually I met Paula, Donna and David and of course Deadlee's mom, Margaret. What an honor.

It is truly humbling when you get so much support from this on-line Twitter thing and then to meet those same people, who have on more than one occasion, lifted me to different doctor visits and procedures.

I would simply post in the morning that I was going to have either a test or chemo and the response was simply overwhelming.

Thanks to Art and everyone else, the list of friends keeps growing and I hope to one day meet everyone.

Early on I also started following @Xeni aka Xeni Jardin. She is an editor for the online Boing Boing Magazine /Blog. She was diagnosed with breast cancer very close to when my colon cancer was diagnosed. She has been very public with her cancer treatments and I have learned so much from the information she forwards online. She is also very accessible on Twitter and while I have never met her I have asked her many questions and she always answers to the best of her knowledge. I really trust her and she has been a huge inspiration.

Like I mentioned, Twitter does suggest following certain people, the whole algorithm thing. So because I followed Xeni, I started to follow two other people with cancer, @suleikajaouad and @AdamsLisa, both amazing women and truly inspirational writers.

As I was going through my chemo and radiation treatments, I would be reading daily about their personal experiences and wondering how they were able to get it together enough to not only write but to write brilliantly. They inspired me to start my blog and to start letting everyone know what exactly I was going through.

It took me almost a year to start writing. By then I was just starting the twelve chemo treatments that would kill my cancer, once and for all. When I started my blog I chose to use Tumblr as my blog spot. I'm not that computer savvy so I needed something that was easy to use and Tumblr has worked fine. It allows you to link and share to your other social media sites.

Once I finish with a story, I have my blog set up so once I publish it, it automatically goes to Twitter and Facebook. That way I'm able to share with friends that don't use both sites.

Also, I hope that my story can reach anyone that might want to talk or share their story with me. Even though we as cancer patients are surrounded by friends and family and they give us their unconditional love and support, having cancer can be a lonely existence. We suffer quietly, in our rooms, we cry when no one is around. We go through worst case scenarios. We wonder what we should do with all our stuff.

Who do we give all those bobblehead dolls to? All those DVD's we bought and now we have the same movies in BluRay. Yes we go there.

We're asked in the hospital to fill out all those end of life forms; wills, next of kin, funeral plans etc. That's our reality. No guarantees.

Don't be shy. Find a support group. Use the internet. Go to Tijuana!

A Million and One Questions About Diet

Right away, after my diagnosis I was asked about my diet. What can you eat? What diet do your doctors have you on? Ummm....no diet. My doctors never mentioned a specific diet. So I don't know if these questions were out of curiosity or that they knew someone who had cancer who was on a restricted diet. I don't know.

I know there were suggestions to what I should eat if I was feeling nauseated. I know they wanted me to eat healthy, lots of protein, stuff like that. But because everyone is affected differently with their respective cancers, I don't think there is much you can do but wing it. That's, of course, during chemo.

During radiation therapy things did get drastically harder. I was expecting the worst to happen during chemo. I expected to lose my hair and to lose a ton of weight. I was mentally prepared for the worst. And if I lost my hair? So what! If I lost weight? Good!

During my third chemo treatment I asked my nurse in the infusion center, "So when does my hair fall out?"

Chemo is every two weeks so we're talking six weeks into treatment and I still had a full head of hair; no hair on my pillow or falling out during showers.

The nurse, Adele, said that sometimes it doesn't fall out. OK. Cool. And I wasn't losing any weight either. My appetite was good but I did cut back on the junk. And I was very lucky that my brother Kevin cooks healthy!

He has a garden in the backyard and grows a good variety of veggies. I still would have the occasional taco and In-N-Out pit stops though. As the fifth and sixth chemo treatments came up, my appetite was definitely down and so was the type of food I was able to eat. Nothing appealed to me which made it difficult for Kevin, who was nothing but a champ throughout this whole ordeal.

I finally told him to just put something in a tortilla and I'd eat it.

Seriously, that's all I could handle. But I never got sick, I never threw up…until radiation!

There was no rest period in between the switch from chemo to radiation. I was very worn out from the chemo after three months of treatment and now I had to endure daily radiation treatments, 28 in all, Monday thru Friday.

And I was connected to a chemo pump 24/7. This is when I started taking the Metamucil.

The radiation was to be focused on my rectum but of course it still would affect that whole area. And because of the unusual nature of my tumor, I was going to be getting an extra zap or two or three of radiation. Sure enough, after my first treatment, I got diarrhea. And I would continue to have diarrhea about twice a week.

Eating was a challenge. Shit, everything became a challenge, especially going to the bathroom. After the first week of radiation all the skin around my rectum was gone. And my rectum became rawer and rawer, so when I pooped, it felt like molten lava was coming out of my ass.

Yes. I cried. Every time.

This is when I did lose some weight. I had a head full of hair and a big old beard too. It was my act of defiance in the face of cancer. Fuck you, Cancer.

After radiation ended, it took about a month before I could poop normally. I still was barely eating but I was getting enough protein to heal. I had to get ready for surgery.

Six weeks after my radiation treatments, I met with my surgeon to discuss the date and the procedure. This is when Dr. Gregory told me I had to have a colostomy. This is when I went into shock. My initial research into what a colostomy entailed was very depressing.

I found a colostomy forum online and started reading what sounded like a horror story for the rest of my life. No popcorn! Laxatives every day! WTF!

Another nurse, Christine, told me she didn't think having a colostomy would be so restrictive. I didn't want to take that chance, so before my surgery I went out and methodically ate everything I loved and everything I thought I would never be able to eat again; burgers

,tacos, burritos, bacon, and popcorn. It was my Farewell to Food Tour. I Instagramed every bite!

After surgery, I woke up and the first thing I did was look to see if I had the colostomy after all. Maybe, just maybe, there was a mistake, maybe I was just having a nightmare and it was all just a bad dream. Maybe the Governor called and I was reprieved. Maybe Not!

There it was, connected to the lower left side of my abdomen: my Dookey Bag. Reality does fucking bite.

In the hospital I was on a diet. My digestive system needed so much help with all the various drugs being introduced into my body, constantly, especially the hard core pain meds. I do have to compliment the hospital food though, made to order. Not bad, three squares a day.

When I came home, Kevin, my mom, Denise and Jeff were there for me, my wonderful familia, trying their best to help put me back together.

What did I eat when I came home? Hard boiled eggs, toast, everything in small portions – Jell-O and fruit cups were go-to snacks. And I was on some very strong meds, still. Vicodin , nausea meds, you know, the good stuff.

Along with all that, I was also taking a stool softener because pain meds make you constipated. I was being visited three times a week by Home Health nurses, all so awesome,

Keith, who I mentioned before, was the main nurse. Dr. Gregory made sure he was in charge of my recovery. He showed me how to change my Dookey Bags. So we developed a cool relationship and would talk about a lot of stuff. But the most important thing that he ever told me was when I asked him about my diet.

I told him that I had read all these horrific things about what I couldn't eat, laxatives and such. Keith had already made a big impression on me the first time he changed my bag because he did it with such speed and professionalism. Wham Bam Thank You Ma'am! And he was done.

His answer was just as impressionable, maybe even more so. He told me, "Just Eat Healthy. You'll be fine."

Sweet! Wow! That I can do. I can eat healthy…sort of. Once in a while. Right, Kevin? Ha! I got this!

Shit Happens

Eating healthy isn't one of my strong suits. I'm a product (or is it byproduct?) of my environment/'hood. That 'hood being in Santa Ana, or as the natives call it SanTana. There are taquerias and burger joints everywhere and most of them are damn good too. But I'm determined to be a model patient and I really need to make this colostomy work well and not have any complications.

My surgery being in late July, my recovery coincided with the NFL season. Being a great friend and my compadre, Francisco, or as we all call him Fran, would come sit with me and watch Thursday Night Football in my room after he would get off work. Fran works for the city of SanTana in the Ivory Tower known as City Hall. He's the Executive Finance Manager. We call him "The Mayor."

On his way to my house Fran would stop off at Sarinana's Tamale Shop and buy a carne asada burrito and a couple of tall cans of beer. I was pretty much bedridden and eating very light. I would watch Fran munch down that burrito and think that I would never, ever be able to eat a whole burrito again, ever! Maybe half…it seemed so huge and all I could think was how I would ever digest that and then it would just end up in my colostomy bag. Yuck. No thanks.

I was trying to heal not only from my surgery but also I had a few complications. Until I was 100-percent, I couldn't start the additional chemo that I needed to kill the cancer that Dr. Gregory wasn't able to remove. Eating mostly protein I was able to completely heal by December and finally start what was to become 12 treatments of chemo and 25 treatments of Erbitux. A long haul and I was very nervous. I had already been through so much. I was feeling good, positive, but still I knew my body had to be weakened by the previous years' worth of treatment.

But by December, my appetite was pretty normal. I could eat a whole burrito. Yay! Again, I was never asked to eat a certain diet. I just followed the sage wisdom of Keith, my ostomy nurse. Eat healthy.

The one thing I could never fully incorporate was exercise. I fully recommend it to anyone going through cancer treatment. If your body can handle it, do it. We're all different.

I was out of work for a year and a half and was never able to do anything other than walk around a bit, at the mall, or at Target. They're pretty big. I became a hermit, a recluse, avoiding people as my immune system became weaker and weaker. I would go grocery shopping either very early or very late, a habit I still keep today. So I gained some weight, everything I had lost plus another 40 pounds.

Not that I was eating a lot, I wasn't going to the all-you-can-eat buffet or anything. I was just not getting enough activity and I was given steroids before every treatment to help with the pain.

The last month of my chemo treatments I wasn't eating much but I did start a new hobby. I started to smoke meat; wings, bacon, ribs, tri-tips, meatloaf, ham. I'm a smoking savant. I love food, always have, always will.

My Mom tells me that when I was six months old her doctor wanted to put me on a diet. She told me that my Abuelito, Pedro Flores, was so mad.

"How can you put a baby on a diet?!" he asked her.

Anyway, I have gotten used to the colostomy bag. Do I have a choice? It's a full-time job.

I always check the bag throughout the day at work. Sometimes it puffs up from gas. I try to empty it as soon as I have a movement. I try to avoid an accident. I keep it clean, all day, every day. But I'm OK with it. I've had a few accidents, and I handle them.

Tell me if you've heard this one...shit happens! Ha!

Fuck cancer!

My Room, My Safe Place

My room is a very small room, with a big screen TV and an old school turntable. It's my sanctuary, my office, my church. My room was so many different rooms at different times during my year and a half of treatment. I realized right away, after I was diagnosed, that I would be spending most of my time in there.

The first thing I did was purchase a 47-inch, LCD, 3D flat screen with a 3D Blu-Ray player. I wanted a Samsung but I settled for an LG and I am very happy with it. I am not a huge fan of 3D but at the time I got a very good deal on Amazon. Pre-tax days, it came out to $1,150 for the TV and Blu-ray player, no tax and free delivery. I was set!

I already had Netflix and a bunch of movies but I mostly watched Netflix. At that time I had never watched Breaking Bad or The Walking Dead and a few other cult TV shows. So I was able to catch up on all these cool programs. Another favorite was BBQ Pitmasters. I love that show! And it gave me a million ideas on how to smoke meats.

Of course, when I wasn't watching TV, I was either going through treatment or just lying there on my bed, feeling the effects of chemo. And like so many people going through the cancer journey, I had a lot of time to think, to pray, to cry. Mostly I prayed and prayed some more. It was a whole other level of praying. I'm a product of 12 years of Catholic school but I like to keep my faith to myself. I rarely share what exactly I believe in. I think it's my business, but if you want to know, I will tell you.

It's a combination of my Catholic beliefs and common sense. I know. It works for me. I have a pretty good idea what's right and what's wrong. I know how to give the benefit of the doubt. I don't judge. Nope. That's beyond my pay scale. I don't expect to go to heaven or hell. I haven't earned either one. There's always room for improvement.

Right.

So now I'm faced with a disease that wants to kill me. I have a tumor that surrounds my colon and then has grown down parallel with my sphincter and comes out my skin on my left buttock. But I'm the lucky one.

The tumor would statistically grow right up into my liver or some other internal organ. Why it didn't I don't know and I'm sure my doctors don't either. My surgeon, Dr. Gregory, told me this was only the second time she had ever seen this in her career. But a cancer tumor is still life threatening and I could sense my doctors sense of urgency.

They came up with a game plan to first kill that tumor and to shrink it. The surgery would take care of the cancer surrounding my colon.

As the tumor shrank and died, that created the most pain that, at that point in my life, I had ever experienced. At that time I didn't have any Vicodin, just over the counter stuff.

One night, the pain was so intense down where my tumor was; the same tumor that was starting to die and to break up into pieces. Yeah, that tumor, it made sure I knew it was dying. It was the kind of pain that makes a grown man cry, the kind that will not subside.

Oh no, this tumor was just getting started. And when all else fails? Start praying. That's all I had. I had to ride out this pain until the next day when I could go see my oncologist and beg for Vicodin, morphine, anything!

So between the tears and sobs I prayed Hail Marys. So many Hail Marys. And then I did something that came out of nowhere. I started to apologize. I was praying and crying and then I started to say I'm sorry.

I'm sorry…

At this point, I had to assume that I had done something very bad to deserve this pain, this cancer. If I had offended God in any way during my life, then I better apologize. And I meant it. I sounded like a little kid, apologizing and crying.

I'm sorry…I'm sorry…but the pain didn't go away.

I had found in myself a new level of humility and from there I believe my prayers going forward would be answered.

Friends have told me that I'm a walking miracle. I want to confirm that, yes. But I would say it was a series of small miracles that added up to the big miracle. Of course I give my doctors, my Dream Team, plenty of credit for their hard work and to all the nurses and therapists along the way.

Still, there is the power of prayer and positive thoughts that many, many friends, family and even people I have never met, sent my way. So many friends would tell me that I was included in their prayer group at Church. It is very humbling to know that in a church or living room somewhere a group of people would be praying for me.

Thank You.

My room was also where, after being sent home after my surgery, the Home Health nurses would conduct their visits. Three times a week they would come over and change my dressings and my colostomy bag, check my blood pressure and body temp. I had so many boxes of medical supplies that I couldn't even see my old school turntable. The visits lasted for four months as I healed from my surgery and a couple of complications.

So much happened in my little room over the year and a half. It was my safe place. I still find myself just staying in my room, reading or watching TV.

And of course, praying.

Robert Gets His Groove Back

The Island of Misfits is real. It exists right in your home town. An injured soldier, a person with a handicap and many of us that have beat cancer. We walk the streets with many various scars. Some of us have lost limbs, maybe an internal organ or have had a mastectomy. You most likely don't even notice us. We are running errands or going to work and generally trying to get our lives back to normal.

Cancer took my rectum and sphincter and some of my colon. But I went back to work and with a permanent colostomy. I will not allow having cancer to alter my life. If I do, then cancer wins.

From the beginning, I took my diagnosis with cancer very personally. If someone was trying to kill you, wouldn't you? Especially when the odds were in cancer's favor?

Returning to work was a first step and honestly, it wasn't easy. But after a year, I can say that I am as productive an employee now as I was before my diagnosis. Last week, I took the next step to getting Robert's groove back.

I'm a pretty normal, male adult. I've been married before but now I'm divorced and have been for about 10 years now. So I'm ready to hopefully settle down again. I know having a permanent colostomy will not be a selling point. I've gotten used to the bag and the constant checking to see if I need to empty it. It hasn't been easy but I don't let that bother me. Otherwise, cancer wins and cancer can go fuck itself.

After my initial six chemo treatments and 28 radiation treatments, and before my surgery, I wasn't thinking about having sex but I'm a guy and I was curious to see if my manhood was still working, especially after being bombarded with all that radiation.

Because of the size of my tumor, my radiologist, Dr. Ash, explained how they had to give me extra doses of radiation, and thank God it worked! And yes, for experimental purposes I was still able to get an erection. I have to emphasize that sex was the last thing on my mind during this period of my life. All I was concentrating on was killing this fucking cancer.

In June 2013, I was given the thumbs up! No more cancer. Back to work, Robert! Hmm...let's see if I can get it up, for experimental purposes of course.

Nothing.

Well maybe it's too soon, right? I've been so focused on everything else. I'll ask my primary doctor for some Viagra, to help out, why not?

Nothing.

Shit!

Ughhh...

Fuck cancer!

I'm not worried. I've been through worse. Fuck, I'm alive. Cancer will not win this battle.

After my surgery, I was seeing a urologist, Dr. Voruzi. He got me through a difficult time; we've been through some tough situations. I make an appointment. I do some research on the various products that are available for men in my situation.

I immediately rule out giving myself a shot to my penis to attain an erection. That's just crazy. But in fact all these options are crazy. But I'm crazy...I firmly believe that being somewhat crazy is what got me through all this. When I realized my hair wasn't going to fall out, I defiantly grew it out, beard and all, just to spite Cancer the Coward.

So here I am in, the urologist's office, waiting for Dr. Voruzi, a little anxious, but I'm totally convinced that I'm doing the right thing. I compare my predicament to anyone that elects to have cosmetic surgery to enhance their breasts or the nips and tucks that can boost one's ego. Also women that have breast reconstruction after mastectomies and that includes the nipple tattoo. I am ready for the next step to regaining normalcy.

I greet Dr. Noruzi as he comes in the patient room and we exchange the long time no see's like two old teammates that went through hell to win the big game. We caught up with my health status, then immediately got down to the nitty gritty.

Can't get it up Doc.

Is it hormonal?

Nope. I've tried Viagra.

Okay, so you must have nerve damage from your surgery.

Bingo!

Here are some options.

We went through a short list of possible solutions. The one I was most interested in was a penile implant. YouTube has great instructional videos on this one. It seemed like something I could live with. When you wanted to have sex you pumped up an implant that was placed in your penis, kind of like pumping up a balloon. The pump was surgically implanted in your scrotum. It took a few minutes to get it fully erect and you were in business. It would remain hard even after ejaculation.

What the YouTube video didn't tell me, which Dr. Voruzi did, was that once you get the implant nothing else can be used…like the penile shots. When they put in the implant they take out the muscle in your penis. That part I didn't like.

So the other option for me was the shot to the penis. Yikes! Dr. Voruzi explained everything that I needed to know. I trust him. I went for it.

Right there.

Right now.

He gave me a shot of what is called Trimix. It's actually three different drugs. There is a Bimix and also Alprostadl, which he recommended but didn't have any in the office. All three come with the risk of a four hour plus erection which means a trip to the ER…which means another needle to the penis.

I'm at the point of no return here. I'm all in! Cut me, Mick! I mean shoot me up doc!

I've been giving myself shots of B12 so I am slightly familiar with needles and their different sizes. The needle that we were going to use is what diabetics use to inject insulin. It's very small, thank God.

He was giving me the "how to shoot up your penis" lesson but I wasn't really listening. I mean, I was but I could only think, "What the hell am I doing?!"

I was lying down on the small bed they have in these cubicles and it didn't hurt at all. He told me to wait about five minutes for the shot to take effect. He would leave me alone.

Think sexy thoughts, he told me.

I just laid there staring up and he asked, are you OK?

I smiled and looked at him, "It's a new world, Doc."

After five minutes, Dr. Voruzi came back and asked if I'd had a reaction. I was watching a YouTube video on penile shots, not exactly sexy thought stuff. I didn't have any reaction yet. Dr Voruzi said, "Okay go home, hopefully it will kick in and next time we'll up the dose."

Thanks Doc.

I left his office and by the time I got up to my car in the parking structure, I had a raging boner.

A hard-on!

Houston! We have lift off!

Okay, enough with the dick jokes, this is a family channel…sort of. I got something to eat and then went home to deal with my, umm, wiener. It stayed erect for a good hour and then after another hour finally went down to normal.

I was worried about the four hour ordeal but that didn't happen. I then did more internet research and found an old chat room thread about the shots. It was all guys that had prostate cancer operations and also had nerve damage. This was a great find. They were all trading their stories about what meds they were injecting, what worked and what didn't work. The bottom line was that this worked for them and they, along with their partners, were happy.

We all struggle with the cards that we are dealt. Some of us fold and some of us double down. Since the beginning of my battle with cancer I have tried to make the proverbial lemonade out of these fucking cancerous lemons. For the most part I've done well. Overall, I am happy. That's what counts.

Fuck cancer. :)

Acknowledgements

Ed. Note: Robert sent out an invitation for a "thank you" dinner and included why he wanted to thank each person. I wanted to include that here as the "acknowledgements" as it comes straight from his heart.

This is an invitation to a dinner party in your honor. My way of saying: Thank You. It will be at Alcatraz Brewery this Saturday, June 15, at 7:00pm. While many friends and relatives helped and supported me the last year and a half, I want to treat you and a few others to dinner. I don't mean to embarrass you or anyone but I'm going to list the guests and the reason why I am inviting you. There's no way that I could say all this without getting emotional so I'm going to put it on paper. Ladies first…

Mrs. Patty Gutierrez – my comadre. When I first started chemo in January 2011, Patty, along with Frank and Chris, offered to take me to my sessions. While Frank and Chris took me a few times, Patty gave me the majority of the rides. I did pretty well those first six rounds of chemo so when I had to do 12 more the first person I asked for a ride was Patty.

Patty is very busy getting my compadre off to work and getting her kids ready for school but she said yes. It meant a lot to me and I always got to chemo and in a great mood too and with a frame of mind to go through the infusion of poison that would kill the cancer and save my life. Thank you, Patty.

Diana Espinoza – her maiden name. Diana has been a friend for many years. Diana is also a cancer survivor. She is a busy mom and works full time for the county. Not only did she visit me in the hospital but she made time to visit me in the infusion center. And because of the Benadryl they would give me, I was not the best host. But she would stay with me and I did my best to be somewhat coherent. But I really appreciated the company. And her Christmas baked goods were pretty tasty. She brought her daughter Rose to the house to deliver the cookies and other goodies. Yum. Thank you Diana, Miss Noble.

Kevin Flores – my brother. Wow. What didn't Kevin do for me? I couldn't have made it without him, that's for sure. In my darkest moments he was always there for me. He took me to my doctor appointments when I couldn't drive myself. Sometimes these appointments would take all day (his day off), but he made sure I got there. He cooked for me. And it wasn't easy, especially when I lost my appetite, he still made me something. And it was always good and healthy. He cleaned up after me. I would make a mess in the bathroom because I was leaking body fluids from the front and back, I was such a mess…and he would mop up the mess.

He helped during one of my worst weeks, when my Foley catheter got blocked twice. The first time wasn't so bad but the second time was just excruciating, with the pain and the anxiety. Waiting for the nurse to show up seemed like forever and Kevin stayed in my room and talked to me and tried to calm me down and I was just glad he was there. He along with my Mom watched me like a hawk. Thank you Kevin.

Frank Martinez – longtime friend (actually tied with Chris Briones). Frank, Chris and I were at a party when we were one year olds. I have the picture to prove it. Right away Frank made himself available to me for rides and he would always invite me to breakfast, at Willowick, of course. But I really appreciated the phone calls from Frank. First to ask how I was and what was I going through or what was coming up and then just to talk about normal stuff. My normal was not so normal and it was good to hear how his girls were doing in school and how his parents were doing. Of course, the Martinez family did save my life by letting Frank bring over an air conditioner they weren't using! Saved my life! And I'm sure if Frank could have taken me to all my chemo sessions and doctor appointments he would have. But when he could be there for me, he was. Thank You, Frank.

Chris Briones – longtime friend (tied with Frank). Besides going to parties since we were one year olds, Chris and I grew up on the same street…sort of. We went to school from first grade through 12th grade. And his mom, Mrs. Briones, just went through, and survived her own cancer. So Chris was ready for anything.

He knew what I was going to go through it and also offered to give me a ride whenever he wasn't working. He would come visit me after he got off work. Even though I didn't drink at that time I was glad when he came over with a six pack and offered me a beer. When I started with the drug Erbitux, the company that makes it sent me a package with four different skin moisturizers but they didn't really work so well. Chris brought me this skin moisturizer that really worked. The postman knows his skin products. Thanks Chris.

Mike Schmidt – School of Our Lady friend! We also went to high school together but I hadn't seen Mike in years. But we're connected and he made sure that if I needed anything all I had to do was ask. His wife is a cancer survivor. He knows how tough it was for her. He took me to lunch a few times and visited while I was in the hospital. And one day I will take him up on his offer to build a brick smoker for me…Thank you, Mike.

John Hernandez – aka Johnny H. From day one John would always call me to see how I was doing. After my surgery I was really down in the dumps. John called me, and I guess he could tell how depressed I was, which for me is unusual. He gave me one of the best pep talks ever. I really didn't see that coming but I really needed it and it really helped me. It made me realize how much John respected me and how well he knew me. I would say it was a turning point in my recovery. I was that depressed. Thank you, Johnny H!

Francisco Gutierrez – Compadre, married to Patty. Fran is very emotional. I didn't know this. The other night at Noble Ale Works I went to use the bathroom and when I came back he was gone. He left a note saying he didn't want to say good bye for fear of getting too emotional. True story. So I won't go too into detail but I will say this: my surgery really left me in a mess. All I could do was lay in bed and watch TV. So Fran would come by on Thursday nights after he got off work and sit and watch Thursday Night Football with me. That's just one of the many things he would do for me. Don't cry, mijo. Thank You, compa!

Carlos Covarrubias – I don't know if Carlos can make dinner. I know he is visiting his family, but hopefully he can make it. Carlos lives in Florida but always either would call or text me to see how I was doing. I appreciate that, even though he's in a whole other time zone, he would find time to call or text. I know he's been trying to get back in California but hasn't had any luck with finding a job. It would be great if he did find a job here. Thanks, Carlos.

Santino Rivera – I know for sure that Santino can't make it but I want him to know how much I appreciate his support. I met Santino before my diagnosis and we would just joke around about stuff, politics, football etc. When he found out I had cancer he sent me two of his books - so spontaneous, just like that. He asked for my address and the next thing I knew I had these books of his poetry. I was floored by the gesture, and the poetry is badass. I took them with me to chemo. And Santino would always send me messages of support. He's a pretty cool dude and I'm sure everyone here will meet him one day and agree. Thanks, brother!

So please enjoy dinner at Alcatraz. These guys have also been great to me the last year and a half. Thank you!

Postscript

Alright! Are you still with me? We did it! We kicked cancer's ass! Woohoo! I told you this book was gonna' kick ass. Was that Robert the Bold or what? Yeah!

I just want to take a quick moment and let you know that one of the goals of this endeavor was for goodwill and charity, the goodwill part being Robert wanting to have his story available to help people in need. I think that if people share this book with those in need of hope, that it will help accomplish that goal. If you know someone in need of an inspiring story it would be amazing for you to share this book with them in the hope that it helps give them some strength or even a shoulder to lean on.

Robert and I have talked about different ways that we can get people to donate money to help people with cancer. We still have a few tricks up our sleeves and are discussing the different ways in which we can make this happen but as a publisher, I want to invite you to take the initiative and donate on your own.

On the few occasions that I travel one of the things that I enjoy doing is donating time and or money to communities in need. I don't always publicize these things and you don't need to either. The amount that you give is of no consequence but that act of giving is.

Simple things like greeting cards, an ear to listen, a pizza delivery, a fist bump, comic books…the possibilities are endless.

There are numerous places to donate and I'll leave that up to you but one of the things Robert talked about was how painful it was to see children endure the pain of cancer. It moved him. It also had a profound effect on me. I would like to see people donate to children's cancer charities if possible.

Both Robert and myself ask that you donate whatever you can, however you can, to a cancer charity or fund in the spirit of helping others and reaching out from boundaries like internet wires and book pages. Let's help heal each other and be there for others.

That's it. Simple, right? But simple things can have a profound effect that many might not be aware of. Let's all kick cancer's ass together!

Also, I wanted to give out the web address for Robert's blog and his Twitter handle so that people can reach out to him if they want to. One of the things he wants to do is mentor people going through what he did.

You can reach him on Twitter at @foxflores and on his Tumblr blog at: http://robertthebold.tumblr.com. Look him up! Say hello and let him know how this book and his story made you feel.

Thank you for your time and for helping support underground books like this.

-S|J|R

www.ingramcontent.com/pod-product-compliance
Lightning Source LLC
Chambersburg PA
CBHW030013290326
41934CB00005B/324